Cancer's Gifts

A Loving Journey
Toward the
Final Chapter

D1528862

Les Whitney

Cancer's Gifts

A Loving Journey Toward the Final Chapter

ISBN-13: 979-8-3605-9983-8

TABLE OF CONTENTS

Preface 9

Introduction 13
    BEFORE THE DIAGNOSIS 15
    THE BLOG 19
    MY FRIENDS 20

CHAPTER 1. January 2019 21
    TAKING THE NEWS 24
    SCAN RESULTS 24
    KEEP ON TRUCKING 26
    THE MEDICAL AND INSURANCE COMMUNITY 28
    LEARNING MORE 29
    PLANNING, PHASE ONE 30
    TESTIMONIAL: BRETT PYLE 32
    LESSONS LEARNED: THERE'S NO SUCH THING
       AS "BAD" NEWS 33

CHAPTER 2. Understanding the Diagnosis 37
    BACK TO WORK 38
    LATE NIGHT MUSINGS FROM THE BLOG FEBRAURY 4, 2019 41
      About mortality: *41*
      About Prayer: *42*
    THE FIRST GAME PLAN 43
    LATE NIGHT MUSINGS FROM THE BLOG FEBRUARY 10, 2019 . . . 45
    THE PET SCAN 47
    THE FALLOUT 49
    TESTIMONIAL: RICHARD FORD 50
    LESSONS LEARNED: NO MAN IS AN ISLAND 51

CHAPTER 3. Brain Surgery 57

STATISTICS 59
BRAIN SURGERY 61
 5:00 p.m. Wednesday *61*
 7:00 a.m. Surgery Day *62*
 1:00 p.m. Surgery Day *62*
 4:30 p.m. Surgery Day *63*
 Day After Surgery *63*

THE GAME PLAN 64
A SECOND OPINION 65
TESTIMONIAL: MATT ERIKSON 66
LESSONS LEARNED: SCIENCE AND SPIRITUALITY 67

CHAPTER 4. Chemotherapy 71

AFTERNOON CHEMO ORIENTATION 74
 4:30 a.m. *77*
 9:00 a.m. *77*
 11:30 a.m. *78*

RECOVERY: SLEEP IS THE NAME OF THE GAME 78
CHEMO IMPACT MONDAY AFTER CHEMO 80
TUESDAY AFTER CHEMO 81
WHAT'S THE PLAN? 82
SECOND ROUND OF CHEMO 89
FEELING BETTER 92
THIRD, FOURTH, & FIFTH TREATMENTS 93
TESTIMONIAL: DAVID SPANN 100
LESSONS LEARNED: CHEMO SUCKS! 101

CHAPTER 5. The New Normal 105

DEATH!?! 106
THE RETREAT 108
CAREGIVERS 111
CHEMO CUTBACK IS CONFIRMED 112
IT'S HEALING FRIDAY AGAIN 115
DRUGS 119
BACK IN THE CHEMO CHAIR 119
JUGGLING WORK AND CANCER 121

TESTIMONIAL: JACK DALY 126

LESSONS LEARNED: NEAR-TERM PLANS, ETERNAL GAINS. . . . 127

CHAPTER 6. Life's Ebb and Flow With Cancer 131

BACK FROM THE ABYSS..................................132

THE CONVERSATION 135

HOLLAND, AUGUST 2019................................138

HAWAII..142

DECEMBER 2019..145

TESTIMONIAL: VICTORIA KORTLANG 146

LESSONS LEARNED: FOCUS ON WHAT TRULY MATTERS......148

CHAPTER 7. A New Normal..............................151

LIVING LIFE IN 2020....................................153

MY BRAIN 155

COVID-19, MARCH 2020, THE WORLD CHANGED!............156

JUST SPOKE WITH THE DOCTOR, MAY 2020.................161

HEALING FRIDAY REACTION VARIABILITY 163

TESTIMONIAL: LISA PAPINI 165

LESSONS LEARNED: PRIORITIZE AND ENJOY
THE OPPORTUNITIES 167

CHAPTER 8. I Continue to Live..........................171

OUR WEDDING ANNIVERSARY...........................171

THE UPS AND DOWNS 172

AND THE BEAT GOES ON................................175

NEW STRATEGY, MORE TESTS 181

RADIATION 183

TESTIMONIAL: SCOTT VON LUFT 185

LESSONS LEARNED: DEATH IS NOT A FOUR-LETTER WORD. . . 187

CHAPTER 9. Radiation Side Effects..................... 191

GLAD RADIATION IS BEHIND US 192

THE STOCKDALE PARADOX 195

THE GREAT MISTAKE — OR THE MEDICAL PROFESSION
ISN'T PERFECT.....................................196

HARD TIMES, MAY 2021.................................198

THE PREDNISONE DEBACLE.............................200

FEELING GREAT! FALL 2021 202

LEGACY 205

TESTIMONiaL: SUSAN SMITH..........................209

LESSONS LEARNED: DO IT NOW... WHATEVER IT IS.........211

CHAPTER 10. 2022 215

BAD NEWS..217

TEMPORARY RELIEF..................................218

JANUARY 21, 2022...................................219

MORE BAD NEWS 220

EMOTIONAL CANCER BUNGEE CORD 221

NECESSITY OF VULNERABILITY........................222

THOUGHTS ABOUT LOVE 223

THOUGHTS ON MY LAST DAYS ON EARTH.................224

UNEXPECTED RECOGNITION 225

MARCH 2022 226

April 2022..228

TESTIMONIAL: MOHAMMAD KHAN 230

LESSONS LEARNED: "THIS TOO SHALL END" 232

Testimonial: Teresa 237

Conclusion.. 241

PREFACE

On a clear December morning, I stepped outside to play my ukulele. The sun was shining but not hot as it normally is in Southern California, and the air was as warm as a cozy blanket. I wanted to relax, kick back, and play some tunes, something I do most days. But this day, something odd happened.

My left hand could not find the right frets, and I couldn't put enough pressure on the strings to make music. This had never happened to me before. My own body wasn't responding to my commands and something that usually came so easy was inexplicably impossible.

I was shocked.

I repeated the process over the next two days with the same results. The rest of my life seemed fine, I had no other physical or cognitive impairments. I couldn't understand what was wrong. I felt completely normal. I've been playing for years. The frustration was mounting. Was there something wrong with the instrument?

That had to be it.

Yes, that had to be the problem. There must be something with the bridge or strings that I couldn't see. It never entered my mind that it could be anything else.

I was wrong.

After Christmas, I sat down to catch up on some emails. Strangely, my left hand still wasn't playing along, not just on my ukulele, but on my keyboard. Suddenly, I could not hit the keys I was aiming for, and even worse, my hand started bouncing off keys when I wasn't looking. With a bit of humor, I thought *it's hard enough to type emails without my hand going off on its own.* Now, for the first time, a sick feeling welled up inside of me. I was quaking with fear. Something was seriously wrong with my hand. First the ukulele and then the computer; I was losing control of a vital body part. It was time to have a doctor look at it.

I thought I might have Parkinson's or perhaps a small stroke or pinched nerve. The doctor quickly ruled out Parkinson's. He ordered a CT scan of my head and neck and, after some pushing, referred me to a neurologist.

On January 15, I met with the neurologist while we were still waiting for the results of the CT scan. The neurologist ordered an MRI with contrast to get a good look at my brain. She was kind and professional but took my information with a concern that spoke volumes. There was no messing around with these symptoms; they were serious.

At 8:30 in the morning on January 16, my world changed dramatically.

My GP called me with the results of the scan. His voice was tempered with a hint of foreboding. My reaction, however, was as casual as one would thank a tollbooth operator.

"Mr. Whitney, you have a mass and swelling in the frontal lobe of your brain," he said.

To which I replied, "Thank you," and then promptly hung up.

I had just been handed a cancer diagnosis.

INTRODUCTION

"Cancer didn't bring me to my knees.
It brought me to my feet."
—Michael Douglas

Thank you for buying or borrowing this book. There are many people I had in mind while writing it. First and foremost are my family, friends, and my dear wife, Teresa. I want her to be able to say to someone many years from now:

"You never knew my husband, but here, you can read his book and get to know him through his thoughts and innermost feelings."

I would love to leave behind some of what makes me *me*. If, in the process of doing that, I can help others, so much the better. The other audience I have in mind are those who are going through a cancer experience themselves. This isn't a how-to book or even a how I did it book. However, by sharing my ups and downs, I hope I can show you that you're not alone.

And, you may improve your life just a wee bit.

If you or someone you know is going through cancer, this book may help give you a fresh perspective and a new clarity that will be uniquely yours. This is not a "feel good" or "inspirational" book, mind you. My experience and perspective are here to simply open the possibilities and perhaps start a renewed sense of living for you or someone you care about.

When I received that phone call and the doctor told me I had a mass on my brain, I didn't know what to think. All kinds of emotions ran through my mind, creating a massive amount of white noise that made it difficult to completely understand what was said to me. I said, "Thank you" and then hung up because I didn't know what else to say. I was in shock. Since then, a lot has happened. It's been a crazy meandering journey, sometimes exhausting, excruciating and painful, sometimes intoxicating, and euphoric. I want to capture it all in the hopes that it will help explain what I was going through in the last few years of my life. And more importantly, how it may make a difference in your life.

The next group of people I am writing this for are those who want to know how to help friends and loved ones who are going through the journey of cancer. I'll say right from the start that everyone is different. What I want from my friends and relatives may not be the same thing your friend or spouse is looking for. I will spend some time going over what I find to be helpful and not helpful, and maybe you can gain insight from my views on the matter.

Cancer, like any illness, creates a new set of challenges for the family and friends of those who have contracted the disease. The powerlessness, the "well at least you have your XXX" statements and a dozen of other awkward moments are part of the journey. I believe I can give you a new perspective on what not to say, what you can do, and even a few nuggets of support you may not realize are important.

I believe that this experience has given me a unique insight into what both life and death mean. Imagine if you had only three years to live. What would you change? How would you live and what would you prioritize to make the most out of such a short amount of time? I'll share the things that make me happy and the wisdom that I've learned along the way.

I'm not a doctor. I'm not even an expert on how to handle a cancer diagnosis. What I am an expert on is myself. This is the story of my journey. I hope that by reading it, you may be able to take some of what I went through and apply it to your own life.

Regardless of if you have the disease or know someone who does, when you close this book, you'll have better insight, a better attitude, and hopefully, a vibrant kick into this wonderful thing called life... the present moment.

BEFORE THE DIAGNOSIS

Like many people, my childhood was rough. Maybe rougher than yours or maybe mine was a cakewalk compared to yours. I only mention it to give you a bit of perspective on how I view the world and what shaped me. I won't dwell on the specifics, because to me, what is more important is how those early challenges created my resilience and drive to succeed.

I wasn't close with my immediate family, but I always made friends wherever I went, however. I rarely maintained those friendships after college, or after moving on from various work environments.

I grew up on a block where everybody was a jock. Kids were outside from early in the morning until nighttime playing sports. I had my group of friends, about eight of us, who all lived next door to one another. We would walk to school together and play afterwards until dark. I was happy. I was having fun.

And I was a horrible student.

One second grade teacher wrote on my report card: *His smile and his charm won't get him far in life, though he thinks they will.* Thankfully, I've managed to prove her wrong. Although most subjects in school were a challenge for me due to my lack of effort, math was always easy for me. For example, I never understood calculus, but somehow I almost always got the answers right.

In high school, I was in the Madrigals, a singing group that was featured on several local broadcast programs. I even sang at weddings! Like many young men, I was carefree and enjoying my life... in the present moment. That concept would soon prove to be infinitely valuable as we'll soon see.

Academically, however, I didn't put much thought into my grades until I met a girl in Madrigals who inspired me to try harder. Dating her for two years, I managed to get straight As as a senior and as an undergraduate in college. This was a pleasant surprise to my teachers and to me, as well.

It turns out I just needed the right motivation.

Being carefree never diluted my drive to succeed and work hard. I started working full time when I was sixteen, and never looked back. I paid my own way through college working at a gas station. At age twenty-one, I got a job at a national grocery store chain stocking shelves from four in the afternoon until one in the morning.

Going the extra yard was a matter of habit.

One summer, the owner of the gas station (who happened to become my stepfather) was injured in a car accident and couldn't work for three months. Although I no longer worked there, I knew I could help. So, I got up at five in the morning, opened the gas station, worked there until noon when I tried to get some sleep, then worked my shift at the grocery store from 4 p.m. until 1 in the morning. The money wasn't great, but the values and lessons learned were priceless: helping others and working hard were their own reward.

I did this the entire summer of my junior year in college.

After college, I held several entry level positions. One notable job was being hired as operations manager of an international manufacturing company. My work philosophy was to always be underpaid. Now, I don't mean that I wanted to work for a stingy person or perhaps Ebenezer Scrooge. I believed I was paid for one job, and I should provide more creativity, more collaboration, more of whatever I could offer beyond what they paid me to do.

One day, I was cleaning out a desk in an empty office and I found a stack of letters-of-credit just sitting in a drawer. Without asking anyone, I began to call the originators of the letters, only to discover that they all wanted to do business with us. I took the company from $40,000 to over a million dollars in exports in a single year. Great news for the company. And, what did that initiative do for me, personally?

I was promoted to VP sales.

As VP, I was able to travel all over the world, which jumpstarted my eternal love of adventure. A few years later, the company was sold and I decided to open my own export company. We transported law enforcement and sports equipment, backpacks and tents, guns, body armor, and handcuffs.

I love telling people that I was an international arms dealer.

Handcuffs and law enforcement equipment aside, I never even owned a gun. Despite enjoying myself at shooting ranges with clients and friends, I never had the desire to own one myself.

For the next 15 years, I was fortunate to lead three different companies. The challenges and success we had over the years formed much of who I am today. Meeting the needs and expectations of all stakeholders while ensuring opportunities, success, and financial wellbeing for hundreds of employees made me well equipped to handle the challenges I faced as my career grew.

I never would have guessed how those lessons would be used for this new challenge.

I became involved in Vistage as a chair and enjoyed it so much, I also began mentoring other chairs. Vistage is a peer group/executive coaching organization where C-level professionals' network and support each other through regular meetings. It's part advanced education, part work group. Guiding these seasoned leaders through the challenges and opportunities life and business placed before them provided a strong foundation for my cancer journey. Many of the people I met there I consider my closest friends.

I was at a Vistage meeting when I had that fateful conversation with my doctor.

I consider myself lucky, despite or perhaps because of my diagnosis. I appreciate life in a meaningful and impactful way. I am awakened to the beauty surrounding me, able to experience the ups and downs of life in a much more meaningful way, and able to appreciate all the wonderful people in my life.

> *"In some ways, cancer has been a blessing... I am awakened to the beauty surrounding me."*

THE BLOG

One of the first things I did after learning that I was about to die, was start a blog. I chose CaringBridge, *https://www.caringbridge.org/*, a website that provides space for people with terminal disease, their loved ones, and caregivers to connect. Through the blog, I was able to keep my entire tribe updated and share both my deeper feelings and my more fleeting thoughts. Over three years, I posted sometimes several times a week, sometimes only once a month. I posted after a particularly painful diagnosis, after trying chemo treatments, and on vacation in Hawaii. I wrote about the meaning of life and the reality of death, and enjoying what time we have left. I opened myself up to such a degree that many of my friends expressed surprise and fascination.

I want to encourage you to visit the blog and maybe post a comment. As of the writing of this book, I have two new lesions in my brain and a 10mm growth on my adrenal gland. I don't know how much longer I'll be around. If I'm able to read and respond to your comment, I will take the time to do so. If it has become a memorial, then your message will mean so much more!

MY FRIENDS

I couldn't write this book without the support of my wife and community.

I met my beautiful, heroic, kind, and generous wife Teresa over forty years ago. She was the first person to show me unconditional love, and one of the few people I have ever shared my heart with. Before I had a network of close friends, Teresa was someone I could rely on to share my life's struggles. She will always be my first thought upon waking in the morning, and my final thought before going to sleep

When I was growing up and all through my early adult years, I didn't have many close friends. I have come to a place of authenticity in my life, partly due to the disease. I am now grateful to report that I have many people supporting me whom I love unconditionally.

You will notice that I use the word "we" often, instead of "I." This is because I truly believe I am sharing my journey with others. We sat down with several of my friends and colleagues who agreed to be interviewed for this book. I am privileged to know many kind, thoughtful, generous people who are also thought leaders and industry giants. I will leave their testimonies in their own words to spice up the narrative.

Thank you to all who participated.

CHAPTER ONE

JANUARY 2019

When the doctor gave me the dire prognosis, I uttered just two words and hung up the phone. It was not done in defiance nor was I being rude.

"Mr. Whitney, you have a mass and swelling in the frontal lobe of your brain," he said.

"Thank you," was all I replied and hung up the phone.

Normally, when a doctor informs you of a mass on your brain with a cancer diagnosis, you are a deer in the headlights. You might have disbelief, shock, anger, sadness, or any number of confusing thoughts, emotions, and tears. I'm sure he was expecting I'd have a ton of questions. At the very least, one would pause a bit and suggest an in-person visit.

I did neither.

I was polite, but unable to process. The numbness removed any emotional reaction. What I heard was not connected to who I was. "I'm the adventuring, healthy guy!" "What does cancer mean?" "Is he talking to me?"

"Thank you," as I hung up the phone, was all I could fathom. My brain was too numb, too shocked, and frankly, filled with foreboding to think clearly.

I didn't ask any questions. And now I had to tell my wife the results. Talk about a hard conversation. I felt embarrassed and foolish when I explained what happened.

Teresa was a trooper. She didn't scold me for not asking questions; she just said, "We got this!"

After collecting my thoughts, I did contact my neurologist who informed me that we should wait for the results of the MRI before getting too concerned. The doctor told us that this type of tumor did not start in the brain, so we had to find where it started. She also scheduled a full body CT scan with contrast to find the origin of the cancer.

"Oh great," I thought, "Not only do I have brain cancer, but this crap originated elsewhere in my body."

I consider myself a person who thrives in the present moment. I enjoy wherever I go and whomever I'm with. But man, we had planned some travel together. Now, all I could think of was that my body was filled with disease and Teresa would have to spend the rest of her life without me. Strangely, I wasn't scared for myself. I've had a wonderful life and know I can roll with anything life throws at me. My true sadness was for Teresa.

I was sad for her and for all the adventures we wouldn't share together.

The "We need to find the origin of the cancer" statement had me more confused and disoriented. Like before, I did not have any questions. I did not feel anxious, sad, or nervous about my body. But the confusion and immobility were palpable.

Waiting was easier said than done. I had the MRI late Thursday night the 18th and was hoping to get the results on the 19th or Monday the 22nd. The Universe, unfortunately, had other plans.

There were no results on Friday the 19th and Monday the 22nd was a holiday for my doctor. The world did not stop for my results, and I did not stop for the world. I had a large conference with Vistage on Tuesday, so I went as planned.

While I was at the Vistage Chair conference, the doctor called.

This time, I arranged for my dear friend, Linda Hughes, to sit with me during the call to make sure I asked questions this time. Teresa was patched in from San Clemente. The results were grim; we knew I had a malignant brain tumor that was 19mm by 17mm in the back of the frontal lobe of my brain. Now the doctor was telling me I had stage IV lung cancer. The way she said it had me believing she was giving me a death sentence.

I just knew I had to get home to be with Teresa.

It's difficult to imagine, but my brain was in such a deep fog, I was unable to process something as simple as turning on the GPS to drive home.

"Where did I park?"

"Which highway do I take?"

I knew I had to go home... like NOW.

All my Vistage friends at the conference pulled together and made travel arrangements to get me home. Without them, I don't know how I would have managed. My thoughts were simultaneously moving at warp speed and slow motion.

TAKING THE NEWS

While many people sink into a strange mix of depression and hope, I/we looked at this as simply another journey in our lives together. We have been through tough situations before and always excelled, so we knew we could do it again. I did not see this new information as a death sentence. Rather, it was simply another item to be managed. I saw the journey as a part time job added to my life. I was fortunate that I chose to transition one of my CE groups to another chair the previous year reducing my workload by 40%. I had planned to use my newfound time for more travel.

Instead, that time would be allocated to this part-time gig...getting healthy.

I saw this journey as being similar to walking the Camino de Santiago (a 500-mile walk in Spain where Teresa and I spent 31 joyful days in solitude and self-discovery). Each day I woke up not knowing where I would be going, what my day would be like or what challenges we would face. I am so glad I walked the Camino and believe it was placed in front of me just so that I would have this perspective.

My goal was clear. Teresa and I would someday walk the Camino de Santiago again, hand in hand with my ukulele hanging from my backpack.

SCAN RESULTS

The second diagnosis of lung cancer was even more shocking than the initial brain tumor. There are hundreds of body parts where cancer can begin. From our bones, organs, skin, and other tissue, the complex web of our systems means blood and cells can transport themselves around quite a bit. Of all the locations possible, one of the most challenging areas is the lungs. The transport and filtering of blood and oxygen is a complex process that is part liquid and gas. So naturally, my cancer began there.

In my right lung.

I am still trying to comprehend that I have stage IV lung cancer.

Which, I have been told, is one of the most deadly and incurable forms of cancer.

This was nearly as shocking as the initial brain tumor diagnosis itself. My brain would not accept "lung cancer." I have always lived a very fit and healthy lifestyle. My diet is full of whole foods, my fitness routine is the envy of my peers, and I never smoked.

Lung cancer?

That made no sense. "Maybe they were wrong?" I secretly said to myself. "No... these guys are good, Whitney. You just wish they were wrong." As much as I tried to deny or justify the origin, it made little difference.

Cancer does not care.

My non-smoking life and healthy living didn't guarantee a cancer-free life, it seems. However, healthy living does matter. Healthy living still improves your odds. Healthy living creates a better life. In fact, as you'll soon see, even though cancer ignored my healthy lifestyle, those habits would become vital as we navigated the journey. More on that later...

We set up an appointment with the neurosurgeon on the following Monday morning and the pulmonary oncologist for Tuesday morning. The anxiety kicked in...

Rather than sit around moping, we decided to go play golf. I was quite a sight playing as my left hand flew off the club almost a third of the time I tried to swing. My golf "handicap" seemed literal as we sliced and diced our way across the green. Luckily, I didn't lose any clubs, but Teresa wisely kept her distance. My left leg started acting up, which didn't do much for my swing. It felt weaker than it normally did and considering the events of the past few days, that had me concerned.

I don't remember the score. Probably better that way.

I was still exercising every day and that was important for my mental health. I didn't want to face a future where I would be limited in my ability to get out and enjoy life. My strength and endurance were being impacted. I got tired after only nine holes which was also unlike me. Cancer is a powerful disease, and it was just beginning to flex its muscles. This was not a fight or a competition, it was quickly becoming a way of life.

Cancer and I were learning to communicate.

KEEP ON TRUCKING

The weirdest sensation began to take hold of me, and I struggled to explain to my friends what it was. The outside of my body didn't seem to know what was going on inside. Here I was, with both lung cancer and brain cancer yet, except for my useless left hand, I felt the same as I had a month ago.

Teresa and I walked seven miles on Saturday and another six miles on Sunday with no strain. Perhaps that was why my anxiety level was low and my optimism was high! I was running off exercise induced endorphins. Don't get me wrong, I knew my diagnosis could easily be a death sentence; I just felt strong and determined to kick cancer's ass before it kicked mine.

I noticed how hard this was on those who were close to me. They were all powerless and felt like they could only provide me with support and prayers. They wanted to do more, and I knew that had to be frustrating. It's one thing to be self-absorbed about my own health, but when my condition impacts others directly, the effects are compounded. When I saw Teresa struggling with these emotions, it broke my heart.

It was wonderful to know I had her support, the support of my family and friends, and the support of everyone following my journey. But in some ways, I was going through it alone. We were all alone with our own thoughts, and only by spending time together and being honest could we help each other get through it.

If you are close to someone with cancer, there's plenty of advice available. People often say and do things they think are helpful, but may be ill-timed, unnecessary, or downright awkward. The bottom line for me was not how empathetic or encouraging a person is. Rather, the acknowledgment of my journey was all that mattered.

Some responses by close family members to my cancer raised my anxiety level. They were traumatized and this manifested itself in them acting as if I was already gone. It felt to me as if they were looking to me to make them feel better or make it all right. Others were so hell bent on making things better, the "You'll get through this" or "You can 'beat' this," sayings often caused me more anxiety as my cancer is considered "incurable" and I felt compelled to explain this to them.

Teresa and I had enough on our plates.

Our strategy was simple. In the interest of managing our journey and removing the collateral damage to others, we avoided them until they could come to grips with my cancer on their own.

This was hard for them and us. However, at the time, it was the right thing to do.

THE MEDICAL AND INSURANCE COMMUNITY

Always healthy, I never had to deal with the medical community before beyond the occasional hiccup. But as soon as I discovered I had cancer, I was thrust into the middle of a bureaucratic nightmare. Maybe nightmare is too strong a word, but it sure felt like it at the onset and I'm sure I'm not alone. Bottom line, the red tape in our healthcare system ranks high on the "could be challenging" scale.

Every scan, MRI, or even first appointment with a specialist required me to stand up and advocate for myself. My first attempts to get more information with specialists were met with, "Our first available appointment is one week or one month out."

While I am generally a very polite and pleasant individual, this was not the time for being friendly and accommodating. With a little pushing, persistence, and help from higher authorities, I put my needs first. I had to make demands. When faced with being dropped into the meatgrinder of our healthcare system and asked to wait, I persistently and politely responded,

"No, we actually have to do this tomorrow."

Moving forward, I met with the neurosurgeon on Monday, pulmonologist on Tuesday, and then a bronchoscopy on

Thursday. The bronchoscopy is a procedure where they run a camera through your nose and then down into your lung. They planned to grab a piece of the tumor and pull it back out. This would give us an opportunity to put a name to my cancer and plan the treatment strategy.

LEARNING MORE

Now that an initial strategy was in place, my desire to not talk to others increased. I was moping around; I was just not compelled to think about anyone else but me. I've learned this is typical of cancer patients in the early stages of their journey. Too many unknowns, too much information, and too much fear and anxiety take their toll. The next day, however, I was all excited about conducting my first one-to-one mentoring session with a Vistage peer since learning about the lung cancer a week ago. The difference in my mood from day to day was astounding. While I could have done without the lows, I was grateful that they weren't all consuming.

What a difference a day makes.

I was also grateful for the love and support I was getting from everyone. My amazing wife Teresa was and is, an absolute rock. Sure, like any mortal, she has her moments, but day in and day out, she was figuratively and literally standing beside me.

This was not just *my* journey; this was *our* journey.

My family rose up and sent me positive vibes daily. I informed them that I was not open to any sadness, just positive thoughts about possibilities and strategies. I knew that they needed to cry and express their concerns. That is normal for people who are connected to those of us with cancer. However, their pain and concerns don't always fit with my mission. For once in my life, it wasn't about helping someone else feel better. My job was not to understand their sadness or console them. I had no issue with them expressing their sadness or concern.

I just preferred that they do it without me in the room.

The love I felt from the Vistage community was nothing short of a miracle. Their guidance, willingness to jump in and help, and moral support gave me the confidence to tackle the challenge. My members often told me their experience with me and Vistage changed their lives. I did not want my diagnosis to change our relationship. While we did set aside time to speak about my cancer, we spent most of our time discussing their opportunities and challenges. Just as before my diagnosis, consulting others is my fuel. It gave me a renewed sense of normalcy during those initial crazy days. Not only did our discussions directly improve their business, they often explained they were looking at my journey to support me in return.

> *"If anybody should get cancer, it's me. I've got the most positive attitude in the world."*

PLANNING, PHASE ONE

The first time we got to see the images of the tumors in the brain and lung was eerie. Reviewing images of these things that were inside my body resembled an autopsy on an alien. The tumor in the brain was the size of an olive. The tumor in the lung was the size of a golf ball. Staring at images of both didn't make me want to mix a martini or play golf.

It felt like I was staring at the mug shot of my killer.

The cancer moved from the lung to the brain and was considered stage IV. That meant surgery to remove the cancer from the lung was probably not an option because it had already metastasized. We would have to count on a different treatment to kill or at the minimum control the cancer in my lung. We needed to determine what type of cancer I had.

A biopsy was ordered via the bronchoscopy.

Results?

"Mr. Whitney, we'll know more after the procedure on Thursday. We'll just have to wait and see."

Wait and see?

One of the most interesting things when navigating cancer is not the diagnosis, but like music, it's the space in between the notes... the waiting. Our minds can fly from worst case to best case outcomes in a nanosecond. What this does to our spirit, attitude, and body is obvious.

Controlling or managing thoughts during the wait is no small order. I found myself walking around our home looking for the best place to put my hospice bed. Not a healthy thought this early in my cancer journey.

The doctor said that they would likely do a procedure known as stereotactic radio surgery on my brain that would use radiation to target the growth. It sounded macabre but it would be less invasive than a drill and Swiss army knife, so I was pleased. We were going to delay the brain work until after the oncologist could come up with a strategy for the rest of my body.

More waiting.

Rational thoughts always came back to put me in check. What other choice did we have? Ramping up my education on cancer involved scores of discussions, reading, and evaluations. While there were disagreements on a few things, there was one item on which we all agreed.

As I was leaving the pulmonologist, I said to her, "This is some bad shit, isn't it?"

She replied, "Yes, this is some bad shit."

At least we could agree on that!

TESTIMONIAL: BRETT PYLE

I met Brett through Vistage. We had many meaningful discussions about cancer, goals and life in general. . I'll let Brett explain in his own words:

My name is Brett; I'm a Vistage chair. I have not been chairing as long as Les. But he was a bit of a legend in our community for a variety of reasons. He did a lot of group launches, establishing new chairs and helping with logistics, so I knew him by reputation. I had not met him until an event called Keepers of the Flame. I can't quite remember the exact year, but it would have been the year he got his diagnosis.

Keepers of the Flame is an event that's reserved for chairs that have been doing the work for at least ten years. I ended up having dinner with him one evening there and I learned of his story. I have to say I was blown away by his attitude. Les is the most optimistic person on planet Earth. He makes Chris Trager (a Pollyanna type character from the TV show Parks & Rec) look like a pessimist. There were some other Vistage chairs that were with him when he got the diagnosis. And these guys said Les didn't miss a beat.

He said, "Oh, that's fantastic. If anybody should get cancer, it's me. I mean, think about it. I've got the most positive attitude in the world and if anybody can get through this it's me."

He went to the doctor, and the doctor said, "Les, I'm sorry."

Les replied, "Sorry? Come on. Let's figure out how we're going to get me 15 more years."

The doctor said, "Les, you don't get it. The cancer is everywhere. We need to talk about how we get you three more weeks."

Les didn't flinch. He said, "Okay, great. Let's start there."

For me, that story just kind of captures what makes Les so unique. He has an unflappable, positive outlook on life. According to Les, anything can be conquered, you just need the right attitude.

LESSONS LEARNED:
THERE'S NO SUCH THING AS "BAD" NEWS

The myth of control is an important concept in business and in life. To a certain extent, we all want to be in control. To be fair, some of us are more aggressive than others in our desire to control. While I reject the expression "control freaks," I would more aptly state I am an outcome-based thinker and doer. ☺ OK... I have a strong desire to be in control. In part, I believe this trait makes for a better leader; provided it is tempered in the right direction and proper environment.

But in a very real way, control is mostly an illusion.

When you are a passenger in a car or flying in an airplane or going under the knife, you are giving up control. A hundred percent fully and completely. You are trusting the driver or the pilot or the surgeon to take care of you, to guide you safely to the other side without messing up.

When we receive what most would call "bad news," part of that name is due to a lack of control. The words we associate with situations, circumstances, people, and environment often look like we are witnesses—not drivers of the outcome. When the term "incurable cancer" was spoken about my body, it felt like I was no longer in the driver's seat.

But that's not true.

We can't magically wave a wand and cure ourselves, but we can find meaning in our suffering. We can also control our reaction to the diagnosis and focus on what needs to be done rather than what can't continue. It may sound trite to state, "The only thing we can control is our reaction to a situation," but the truth lies much deeper.

Before we can be mindful of our attitude, we must begin with acceptance.

I have cancer, and I am in for the struggle of my life. I may die soon. I am 99% sure that cancer is the thing that is going to kill me. So, why would I expend any energy or thoughts to the contrary? That single aspect of my condition (cancer is going to kill me) can be set aside.

I don't need to think about that specific item anymore. Done.

With that area on the back burner, what do I do? How do I adjust my attitude? What dreams should be adjusted?

When you set aside a major element like that, something magical fills the void.

Clarity.

As soon as I put the manner of my demise on the shelf, I could focus on how I wanted to spend every day going forward. I could focus on this hour, this moment, this very second.

Being "present" is another one of those trite terms. However, when the "big one" (death) has been put on the agenda, becoming crystal clear and living in the moment truly is one of the many gifts that cancer has brought to me. I know it sounds kind of silly or perhaps overly stoic. But, the title of this book is spot on accurate.

My cancer gave me clarity and presence.

More on that later...

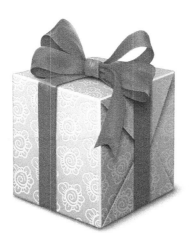

THE GIFT OF DIALOGUE

If I could make one suggestion to anyone who has a friend or family member dealing with a life-threatening disease, it's to engage with them, talk with them about their mindset and emotional state, help them understand their own emotions, and allow them to express their state of mind without judgment or commentary.

I can't imagine how people who are walking a cancer journey alone endure and survive. I know that when I am faced with *difficult* news (notice, I didn't say "bad news") that I will have the support of my community. They will be there with prayers, ideas, cards, notes, and most importantly, with their love.

Conversation is the one thing we can all bring to the table. I know that I am not looking for answers from my family and friends. I want their curiosity and their empathy. Sharing stories of personal experiences with cancer is helpful. Most valuable are open-ended questions about what I am thinking, feeling, and believing about my situation. These questions allow me to clarify and help me understand my own emotional journey.

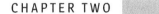 CHAPTER TWO

UNDERSTANDING THE DIAGNOSIS

The bronchoscopy went well. I loved all the attention I got in the hospital while they prepared me; I really felt the love. My doctor was able to get a good sample from the lymph node but struggled to get into the lung deep enough to get a sample of the tumor. That said, the sample from the lymph node was enough to identify the cancer. I still needed to speak to a pulmonologist and then an oncologist to learn what it all meant. The more we learn, the more is unknown. Another cool note is that my neurosurgeon went out of her way to stop by to check on me while I was coming out of anesthesia. Again, I felt the love while she awaited her turn to play with my brain.

Whew! The amount of information and education makes me feel like I could curate content for WebMD.

There are good and bad side effects of this journey.

Good: Teresa and I cannot get enough of each other. We are constantly touching, hugging, and holding each other tightly. We are definitely in this together.

A Twilight Zone Moment

Do you recall the twilight zone episode where doctors were trying to help a woman look normal but her faced was wrapped in gauze the whole episode until the final horrible reveal? They slowly pulled the gauze off the woman's face and were shocked at what they saw: a stunningly beautiful woman. The doctors and nurses, all in masks, were visibly disappointed and stated the surgery was unsuccessful.

Then, the doctors' and nurses' masks came off and they all had the faces of pigs with distorted faces and bulging lips. When we got our MRI results back, the stress had taken its toll. Unfortunately, Teresa looked like one of those doctors or nurses with half her face and lips swelled up beyond recognition.

She's the most beautiful woman in the world to me, of course. We all have a bad hair days. This was hers.

BACK TO WORK

After about three weeks, I had my first full workday since the diagnosis. It was refreshingly great to be back. I felt valuable, useful, and needed. I am truly blessed to do work for Vistage, where I get to know my members better than almost any other person in their lives. We talk about fears, hopes, dreams, challenges, beliefs, etc. at a deeply personal level.

Oddly, my experience allowed us to explore the fears around my illness and their personal relationship with cancer in a safe, comfortable, and loving context. I'm reminded of the quote, "being listened to/heard feels so much like love, I cannot tell the difference."

I met with three people that day for two hours each and drove about 100 miles between meetings. I ended the day tired but full of life. The next week I was back full bore with thirteen meetings over four days (hoping that doctor appointments would not force me to change my schedule). I really looked forward to being with my members as I felt in control and it took my mind off of other things.

I love them all.

> *Every one of us has cancer cells trying to take hold at some point or another in our bodies. For the most part, our immune system takes care of it.*

When I finally spoke to the pulmonologist, I got the proverbial information overload. All the assumptions regarding my cancer were bad, but the news was positive. First off, the surgeon who took the biopsy was not optimistic that he gotten a good sample. We were pleased that he did get a sample good enough to identify the cancer, otherwise they would have had to cut into my brain or lung to get a sample. We were disappointed that the sample was not large enough to test for targeted therapy, a less common though much more effective cancer treatment.

Medical Nerd Moment

I have a common form of lung cancer called adenocarcinoma. The cell structure is moderately to poorly differentiated with "mid-high-grade behavior," i.e., the movement or spread. What this means is that my cells have mutated well beyond their original shape quickly. My right hilar lymph node has cancer as well. The plan described here is not for medical advice or diagnosis. Rather, I share it here so if you or someone you care about is going through this, you'll have a better idea on the depth of knowledge you may want to be prepared for. Also, do yourself a favor and don't overdose on the internet. Too much information can be as problematic as too little.

The plan was complex with many moving parts.

Below were my thoughts at the time. My neurosurgeon could proceed with her plans to do proton radiation surgery (SRS) on my brain to eliminate the mass. This process takes two beams of radiation focused on the edges of the tumor. The beams unite and instantly kill the tumor while not hurting the healthy cells. It is a long slow process. The plan was to coordinate with all the other specialists and work it in and around the other treatments. I had no doubt that it would kill the brain tumor. My primary hope was this procedure gets me back to playing the ukulele and not damage anything else.

1. Before investigating all the options, the doctors ordered a PET scan of my entire body to see if the cancer had set up house in any other locations. If the scan was clean, then all options were on the table. More choices is always a good thing.
2. If the cancer was limited to the lungs and brain, then we hoped there would be a chance a thoracic surgeon could remove the tumor from my lungs. Due to my overall good conditioning, the doctors believed I would be a candidate for this. I had a pulmonary

stress test scheduled for the following Tuesday that I passed with ease. This is serious surgery but, coupled with the brain surgery, we could start the chemo with a fairly clean body. Unfortunately, the doctors determined that lung surgery was not an option. Limited options is not a good thing.

3. One upside is that my cancer, adenocarcinoma, is one of the most well-researched cancers out there. That translates to a wide variety of alternative treatments. As with all cancers, there are many mutations. Most of these mutations have highly targeted remedies that are less invasive than full bore, IV drip chemo treatments. Some are as simple as a pill, still hard on the body but less invasive. I was so optimistic and filled with hope that we would qualify for targeted treatment. Sadly, we did not have a good enough sample and were told we had to rely on more traditional treatments. This was an emotional setback for both Teresa and I.

Sidebar: I am sure the medical accuracy of all I've written is not perfect. It is my interpretation of what I heard from the pulmonologist. In addition, always take someone with you to doctor appointments. I found I could not hear and comprehend everything myself.

LATE NIGHT MUSINGS FROM THE BLOG
FEBRAURY 4, 2019

About mortality:
People tell me they are impressed with my mindset and my "one step at a time" attitude I have. I am glad I can be this way. That said, my mortality does cross my mind at times throughout the day. We are all going to die someday, we just don't know when. My time could be 30 years from now or next year. I suspect that whenever it happens it will be cancer related now that I know my body is susceptible to cancer.

What is truly fascinating is the cognitive bias known as the Frequency Illusion or the Baader-Meinhof effect. Now that I know I have cancer, all I see are articles, stories, headlines, and news reports about people dying from cancer every day. This awareness doesn't elude me but it doesn't define me either. For brief moments I allow myself to wonder, "Is this it?" "Are we on a no-win path?"

Sure, I'm positive. Yes. I have a "one step at a time" attitude. But, I'm human. These fleeting moments of "Oh crap, I'm dying sooner than I planned" happen. Nobody is immune from having them.

I've lived my life intentionally for the past fifteen years with the personal mission statement, "Help others achieve the greatness within them." I've been blessed to be successful in this mission in many ways throughout the years, and I intend for my current journey to help others endure and thrive in their similar journeys. This gives me great peace as we walk this road of uncertain distance. I will continue to strive to be a beacon of hope and a conduit to personal greatness for those I am fortunate enough to touch in my life.

About Prayer:
I am not a religious person. I do believe there is an energy or a force that unites all of us. I can feel it now more than ever. Your prayers embrace me every moment of every day. I can truly feel it. Knowing that I have Buddhist, Hindu, Muslim, Sikh, Jewish, and Christian prayers coming my way gives me so much strength. My entire being is surrounded by an aura of love, hope, and happiness because of your prayers. Please keep the love and prayers coming for Teresa and I and for all the people suffering from life-threatening illnesses.

Maybe my religion is love...

THE FIRST GAME PLAN
Our team decided to take a simultaneous, two front approach to defeating or controlling our disease. The lung cancer is the evil demon in our saga and had to be addressed post haste. Since it had moved through the lymph nodes to the brain, we knew those evil cancer spies were lurking in my blood stream, seeking out targets to attack so we had to get after them quickly.

I had the PET scan set for February 11, 2019. This scan looked at the cellular structure to see if there are any other minute areas that the cancer had taken residence. We didn't think it had set up camp but needed to find out to be sure. I met with a pulmonary stress specialist to determine if I could handle lung surgery to remove the mass (as if anyone would doubt that I could handle surgery, I'm super Les!

LOL). I met with the pulmonary oncologist/thoracic surgeon to set the surgery date (if no other mass found).

While all this is happening, my biopsy samples were in a lab somewhere being evaluated to see if highly targeted chemo therapies can more effectively kill my strain. As mentioned before, we were hoping for targeted therapy because it is more effective and less stressful on my body. We were hoping to have a good feel for all of this by my birthday on February 24.

So much hoping.

So much waiting.

So much stressing.

While all this crazy, chaotic, confusing, and scary activity felt like months or years in this cancer journey, all of this transpired in just over a month since I noticed the loss of use of my hand.

Life can be turned on its head so quickly and in such a profound way.

While the brain tumor was secondary to the lung cancer, we chose to seek and destroy it right away. The doctors believed it was more deadly in the near term. The radiation oncologist met with my team and created a plan of action. We decided to do an SRS procedure (stereotactic radiosurgery also known as proton surgery).

Much had to happen before the surgery which I will go into more detail later. First, we needed a highly precise MRI. I understood this to mean I would spend over an hour in the tube (I'm a little claustrophobic, therefore a little anxious). The MRI does two things. First, it will show us if there are any other micro tumors in the brain that need to be destroyed. The doctor said he could get up to fifteen of them if necessary. I doubt we will find any but it's important to be diligent. The second thing the MRI does is provide the road map for the computer added surgery.

> *Fifty-eight percent of Americans will visit a doctor/hospital with some form of cancer in their lives. It just shows us that the survivors outnumber the others by a huge number. I'm looking forward to the day I have tattooed on my ass, "I am a cancer survivor!"*

The next step was for me to go in and have a mask molded around my face—a tight mask. I mean really tight; did I say I was claustrophobic? With this mask on I am bolted to a table to do another CT scan to provide the directional guidance system for the computer. I get a break at this time while the radiation oncologist, the neurosurgeon, and two physicists program the surgery. Then they will place my mask on a plastic dummy and test. After all this, I will come in, get fitted into the mask, get locked into the machine and.... ready set go, they'll push the bottom, walk away, and have a coffee while the machine works its magic. The doctor said I could tee it up and play golf the morning after the surgery. Imagine that: brain surgery and then golf the next day.

LATE NIGHT MUSINGS FROM THE BLOG
FEBRUARY 10, 2019

It's half past midnight and I'm sitting alone with my thoughts, unable to sleep. This is the second night in a row. I haven't been thinking about the cancer. The thoughts that are rattling inside my brain and keeping me from falling asleep are more about who I am and how I think about who I am.

I am not a victim.

Period. End of story.

This is my primary and unshakable belief.

What is happening to me is exactly what *should* be happening to me based on my natural, unique genetic makeup honed from thousands of years of evolution, plus the infinite number of choices (conscious, subconscious, and unconscious) that have led me to this moment. My health, my mindset, who I am, and who I am now are the natural conclusion of my nature and my response through life to the unique stimulus only I have experienced. Many would say this is natural design. I choose to say it is a natural consequence of my life so far.

In other words, I am not a victim.

Why is this important to share?

Because I am not afraid of the outcome of our cancer journey. We are going to get the result we are going to get. Our results will be a product of who I am today and the choices we make moving forward. We choose to focus on those choices, take in the journey with all its ups and downs, joys and sorrows, happiness and fear. Staying focused on the next step while embracing the wonders of our community is how we will continue to walk our Camino.

One important choice I am making at this point, is that I am placing a great deal of importance and value in the upcoming PET scan set. This scan will check out my cellular structure to find any other cancer outposts throughout my body (remember cancer is flowing in my blood looking for places to set up residence). If clean, I believed I would have many more and better options. The problem is, I don't know how much of what I believe about the PET is true and how much I've made up in my active little mind. All these appointments, differing opinions, confusing information on the internet, and my lack of understanding of cancer has me creating scenarios in my mind that may or may not be true.

I was reminded by my friend Rachel Copley-Kornman of the Stockdale Paradox, named after Vice Admiral Jim Stockdale:

"You must retain faith that you will prevail in the end, regardless of the difficulties. AND at the same time you must confront the most brutal facts of your current reality whatever they might be."

My resolve was to respond to adversity differently, confronting reality head on, and emerging even stronger.

THE PET SCAN

We had high hopes for the PET scan and the pulmonary stress test. If the PET scan came back with no more cancer and the pulmonary came back that I was healthy, surgery was supposed to be an option for the lung cancer. Well, the PET scan came back as clean as it could be with the detail it showed. The pulmonary test was a piece of cake soooo... We were all good, right?

Wrong!

Our pulmonary oncologist was not impressed.

"The cancer has already leaked!" he said. "It won't make a difference if we remove it from your lung, it's done its damage."

How is that for a kick in the gut?

"So, what's the plan?" I asked.

"First, we take care of the brain tumor on February 21, and then we start chemo on February 27," he replied. "Which type of chemo is still to be determined, but at least we have a modified plan." To be honest, my desire to learn about the different types of chemo, its usage, and side effects were now becoming a sideshow. My thirst for knowledge was quenched.

I just wanted to get started.

I asked him about lifestyle during the treatment and after we kicked the cancer to its knees. "Can I travel? What will our days be like? How will this impact my work? And of course, how do we deal with the side effects?"

He was very cautious; talked about the many potential side effects and told me we were going to focus on "quality of life" during the next few months. "We will make adjustments, if necessary, to ensure your days are good."

"Adjustments?" I croaked.

"Worry about the near-term impact," he advised.

"Not me," I said, "While I realize I could be dead in a year, I'm working for five to fifteen more good years. I can suffer in the short term!"

You should have seen the look on his face: major constipation to say the least.

"What is that look all about?" I asked.

"Well, we should talk about this," he began. "You see, the average life span of someone who has your cancer that has moved to the brain is six months. Once in the brain, it tends to return."

Now that kick was a little lower than my gut!

Teresa and I just stared at each other.

Not a word.

Not a tear.

We simply froze and struggled to absorb the constraint of time like a boa constrictor eating a hog. We nearly choked on his version of our calendar.

Everything changed in that moment, yet in a strangely peaceful way, everything remained the same. Certainly, we needed to reevaluate our priorities going forward. What was important to us? Would we be the exception to the rule? How could we make sure our affairs were in order for when I died? There was so much to deal with in such a short amount of time. It was informational and emotional overload.

THE FALLOUT

Teresa and I spent about an hour hugging and talking after the meeting with the doctor. I think it just took a bit of time to process what we heard and bring it back to our reality.

I reflected on the message. The doctor was telling us he could arrest the lung cancer through the various therapies, and we could destroy the current brain cancer with surgery. What we could not control was whether or not the cancer returned to the brain to take up residence in a non-operable location.

For whatever reason, chemo does not impact cancer in the brain. Bottom line, this is an "if" scenario, not an inevitability. So, we prepared to move on! Regardless of the outlook, the vision is five to fifteen quality years of adventure.

We would have options about how aggressive we wanted to be with the chemo. The tradeoff was current quality of life vs. longevity of life. What time could we buy with each option and at what cost?

> *I was not into living to avoid dying,*
> *I was into living to ensure good living*
> *going forward.*

If I was confident that very aggressive, miserable treatment would buy many good years, that would be one thing. However, if the same treatment would only buy me two months, I would not be so excited.

I had never felt so centered on myself. For the first time in my life, *I* was the priority. I felt surprisingly good about that. I remained focused on healthy eating, exercise, and time with the people I cared about. It was necessary to maintaining my mental state and stay in what was sure to be a long-term fight.

TESTIMONIAL: RICHARD FORD

Richard was a member of my Rotary Club. He had an honesty and an enthusiasm that brought out the best in me. Here are a few thoughts he shared about our time together:

> *I wondered how I could incorporate Les's enthusiasm and his interest and his curiosity about everything. He used to say, "Maybe you're not looking at this situation the right way. Let's discuss other options you might consider." He had a lust for travel and for life that was unmatched.*
>
> *The fact that he's writing this blog fascinates me, because there's just not a chance in the world that I would be as open as he is with what he's going through. It's raw, and it's mesmerizing. At the same time, it's not surprising that he does it because of his exuberance.*
>
> *As a result of following his journey, I try to be more present. I think we need to go out and experience life. From everything that he's done, it just kind of opens a door saying, "Look stupid, there's so much out there, you're just not paying attention."*
>
> *We're in the stages of planning retirement. There was nobody in my family who did anything big in retirement. We're going to sell the house and buy an RV. We're just going to go travel for however long we can travel. I don't have anybody in my life who's ever done that. And I've typically been more of a follower than a leader and this isn't leading anything, but it's doing something that is new and adventurous. I like to think that Les showed me it could be done.*

LESSONS LEARNED: NO MAN IS AN ISLAND

"No man is an island" is an old adage that means no one can live alone. We know we're social creatures, we organize ourselves into families, communities, states, and nations. We develop ideas about behavior that everyone agrees upon, and if we're very lucky, we fall in love.

This is never more important than when you find yourself faced with the impossible. Death is coming for you or someone close to you, and you need to know how to deal with it.

- How can you put one foot in front of the other when you can see the end of the path?
- How can you find the strength to build a legacy that will endure?
- How can you comfort yourself while going through the most intense, trying, expensive, exhausting ordeal ever?

The answer is elegantly simple: community.

I want to emphasize my great appreciation for the love of my family and friends. It fills and strengthens me in so many ways. These last few years spent among my peers in the Vistage community have made me feel cared for beyond words. It reminds me of the *Wizard of Oz*, when the Wizard told the Tin Man, "A heart is not judged by how much you love, but by how much you are loved by others."

Because of my community of friends, I am rich indeed.

I am writing this book for two different people, those who have cancer and those who have a loved one with cancer. You have a long battle ahead! It can only be made easier with support, well wishes, and most importantly prayers. If a loved one is suffering, please keep the energy flowing and the prayers coming—they are appreciated. If you are suffering, don't remain silent. People are often uncomfortable facing death and don't know what to say. A single direction from you will make them feel useful and will help them help you.

We are so fortunate to live in this period in history with all the medical advances. Add to the scientific miracles a strong community and you will have a much better chance of survival. There are dozens of examples of loved ones advocating for their sick parents, grandparents, and children. Chemo is exhausting. It takes a toll both physically and mentally. The community can provide direction and energy to continue the fight.

I'm amazed at the community that has gathered around Teresa and I. The love, the support, the articles and videos, the willingness to drop other things to be available to us has been inspiring. Then there is the micro-community of fellow cancer patients, cancer survivors, and cancer care givers many of whom we were unaware that had blazed the trail in this journey before. Sharing stories and emotions with them seems to ease the load for both Teresa and I. Our friend Marilyn Murphy and husband Scott visited with us early in our journey. Marilyn recently was deemed cancer clean after a 2-year battle with stage IV ovarian cancer. Discussing the shock of diagnosis, the resolve, the amazing support of our community, and the importance of mindset gave Teresa and I both peace and resolve.

I know that the outpouring of love and support is sincere. I am also aware that this journey is more of a marathon than a sprint. As the updates spread out, as the treatments become same old stuff just a new day, and as our community becomes engrained in their own lives, Teresa and I will have to be more intentional about asking for help and support. I know the support will be there, we just have to be open to it, seek it, and maintain our gratitude for it. One of the things that all the pilgrims would say when faced with challenges while walking the Camino de Santiago is "the Camino will provide." I am confident as we walk this latest Camino that "our community will provide." Thank you for being here for both of us.

I'd also like to take a moment to talk about support for caregivers. Teresa needs as much if not more support than I do. Reaching out and allowing the caregivers to talk openly about the experience, allowing them to express feelings, fears, hopes, etc. that may not be appropriate to share with the patient is so meaningful. My dear friend Craig recently lost his wife to cancer. While she was sick, several couples got together to pull him away from the environment. While one spouse assumed the caregiver role, the other spouse took him out of the house for several hours so that he could work on his own health. This "outsourcing" of care can be extremely valuable to care givers.

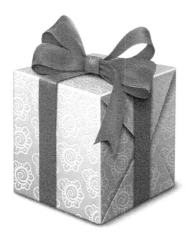

THE GIFT OF RECEIVING

We'll get to the gift of giving in a bit.

First, the extremely obvious gift of receiving. On the surface, receiving a gift is, well... a gift, of course! However, when you peel back the layers of the onion, there is more there than meets the eyes (teary or not with that onion).

Like all Vistage chairs and many of the business owners I've been fortunate enough to work with, we thrive on giving. It's our fuel. Serving others from a leadership perspective builds our worth, value, and self-esteem. In some extreme cases, people who are abundant givers have a difficult time receiving. "Oh, you shouldn't have" or the awkward silence when an unexpected gift of time or service is given to you.

We often don't know how to handle receiving.

One of the many gifts my cancer has delivered to me is my newfound balance of giving/receiving. I'm not a taker by any stretch of the imagination. But the ability to receive had been refreshed and rebooted in my operating system. Looking someone in the eye and accepting and acknowledging their gift (no matter how large or small) is important... not just to me but to the giver.

When faced with new or overwhelming gifts, accept them with grace.

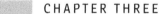 CHAPTER THREE

BRAIN SURGERY

It was my first Vistage meeting since my diagnosis. Fifteen high-powered executives in a room all day to share life experiences, explore ideas to improve their businesses, and engage with a world-class speaker. It felt so good to be back in the saddle, leading my group. To get back in the saddle and do what I was born to do is a feeling that is indescribable. And now, after the past few weeks of what I had been through, I had to do something even more impactful for my members.

This would not be a typical meeting.

We began with a "feelings wheel." Members were presented with about 100 feeling words to help each person share their true emotions when it came to this battle with cancer. Each person shared their feelings about how my cancer was impacting them personally, their past experiences with cancer, and how my cancer caused fear or concern in their own lives. They explored how my cancer impacted their relationships with their families.

I asked three questions to be discussed exclusively using feeling words. The questions were:

1. What feelings are you experiencing around Les's cancer?
2. What feelings does Les's cancer bring up when looking at your own life?
3. How do you choose to move forward? What is possible?

It was a raw, vulnerable, tear filled, loving hour and a half conversation. How beautiful that we could share in such a powerful way! Two people said that they thought the conversation would stay with them for the rest of their lives...and these were the youngest ones!

Full disclosure: no matter how hard I work, how well I eat, how effective my treatments are, the cancer could return to the brain to an inoperable place and...game over.

Through many tears, we were able to share and feel:

- What if it was me, and not Les?
- How would this impact my family and friends?
- How will my life be different if Les can no longer be in it?
- How has my life changed because Les has been in it?

The emotions were raw, the hugs were bold, and the courage compelling. I thanked each of them for their vulnerability, their strength, and their willingness to love each other and me so deeply.

STATISTICS

Fun note: Friday before brain surgery was the day for my mega MRI. I spent the first part of the day relaxing, meditating, and preparing so that I could lie peacefully during the procedure. My doctor gave me an anti-anxiety pill to take half hour before. I took two! The MRI tech took me in, and I was ready. I laid on the table where he injected me with the contrast fluid and rolled me into the machine. It started pounding and whirring around me, but I was ready. I put myself into a peaceful state and five minutes later...he pulled me out and turned off the machine. Apparently, this mind-mapping process for my surgery is the world's shortest MRI.

The burden was then on Teresa to care for a drugged up, completely relaxed MRI wimp.

We were upset after meeting with the pulmonary oncologist a week prior. His comments just seemed to remain in the backs of our minds. So, I decided to look up lung cancer survivability on Google...here's what I found:

"The lung cancer five-year survival rate (18.6 percent) is lower than many other leading cancers, such as colorectal (64.5 percent), breast (89.6 percent) and prostate (98.2 percent). The five-year survival rate for lung cancer is 56 percent for cases detected when the disease is still localized (within the lungs). However, only 16 percent of lung cancer cases are diagnosed at an early stage. For distant tumors (spread to other organs) the five-year survival rate is only 5 percent. More than half of people with lung cancer die within one year of being diagnosed."[1]

That was sobering! Since my cancer spread, the five-year rate averaged 5% and the one-year rate was 50%. Now the good news: only 15% of lung cancer patients never smoked. My clean lungs should be a big factor moving forward. Also, very few cancer patients were in my peak physical condition. At the time, I had similar conditioning to a healthy 45-year-old (I turned 64 that year).

My support community was also key. The daily prayers, affirmations, love, guidance, and support could not be understated nor underappreciated in their impact on my health. All said, I put my odds at 80% to be around for one year and 25% to be here in five years.

All my life I've worked to improve, to just become a little better, a little wiser, a little stronger. Funny how mindset changes. Now the goal of all my activities is to "prolong" my life. That's the word the doctors use, the literature uses, and, therefore, I will use. Prolonging life means to me having a good life for the rest of my life. It means to continue to live my mission, to appreciate every moment, every interaction, every person I touch. It means not being defined by the harshness of chemo, but to persevere through the tough times and make each day as normal as possible.

Gratitude, happiness, and joy are the feelings that flow through me every moment of my journey. I did not write after my group met on that Thursday because I just wanted to sit with and be embraced by the love and caring that I felt all day long on both Wednesday and Thursday.

So, what happened?

I was also looking to maximize those surplus moments. We were joining our close friends for a night at Pelican Hill and a round of golf on Sunday, where many friends were getting together to celebrate my birthday. Teresa and I intended to take advantage of every surplus moment we could during our cancer journey. I had a fantasy that if I could find a three-week window without treatment, I would take the American Airlines around the world trip (one way around the world) to visit as many new places as possible.

BRAIN SURGERY

Stereotactic radiosurgery (SRS) uses many precisely focused radiation beams to treat tumors and other problems in the brain, neck, lungs, liver, spine, and other parts of the body. It is not surgery in the traditional sense because there's no incision. Instead, SRS uses 3D imaging to target high doses of radiation to the affected area with minimal impact on the surrounding healthy tissue.

Like other forms of radiation, SRS works by damaging the DNA of the targeted cells. The affected cells then lose the ability to reproduce, which causes tumors to shrink. SRS of the brain and spine is typically completed in a single session.

5:00 p.m. Wednesday

I was wrapping up my day's work, getting ready for a relaxing evening before people started shooting radiation beams into my brain the next day. Interestingly, I hadn't given a moment of thought or concern to the procedure. I knew it was going to be a long day filled with anxiety. The idea of being bolted down to a machine with a mask on was a little intimidating. I anticipated using the anti-anxiety drugs a couple of times during the process. My sister and brother-in-law would join us for the day, hopefully to relieve some of the stress on Teresa. The only preparation that evening was to take the anti-seizure medication to mitigate the risk of seizure from all the damage they will be doing inside my brain.

I made two requests of the doctor:

1. Get me back to playing the ukulele, and
2. If you can find the right spot in my brain, help me sing better.

I hope to make a recording of playing and singing in a month so that the world can judge his effectiveness.

7:00 a.m. Surgery Day
I went to the gym for an hour-long workout before heading up to the hospital to start the procedure. I decided to maximize every healthy moment I had starting with that procedure. It was time to check in and have my mask made.

1:00 p.m. Surgery Day
The mask was completed at 9:00 a.m. and the CT scan to map me in the mask was done. The mask is a plastic mesh that is molded tightly around my face with about a dozen screw holes so that I can be bolted to the table.

I was finished with all the preliminaries and had to find a way to fill six hours before the surgery. What to do? I decided to be decadent. I enjoyed a pedicure and a manicure and afterwards, headed into a movie theater to watch a movie to pass the time. It was all part of my new mantra: *Maximize every moment!* It would go down in history as the most bizarre surgery day ever!

4:30 p.m. Surgery Day

The surgery was complete and an apparent success! They told me they got it all and there was only one tumor in the brain. The process took about 30 minutes. My head was locked in tight, and the machine moved around to target the various angles. My head felt a little swollen afterwards but that was about all.

They loaded me up with a heavy dose of steroids to keep the swelling down and had me on anti-seizure medicine for a week. They also didn't want me driving for a week in case of seizure. It was hard to believe that I was right back to my normal life so soon after having brain surgery!

Unfortunately, I got some less exciting news right before I walked into surgery. All the biopsy tests were complete, and I had none of the cancer markers that would allow a more focused, chemo pill-based therapy. Instead, I would have to suffer the heavy juice. Not to be deterred, I decided to double down my focus on eating, exercise, positivity, immunology, and everything else that I could control. The real game was about to begin with chemo the following week. The surgery was just an appetizer.

Day After Surgery

We were up at 4:15 a.m. as usual and in the gym by 5:00. Pretty much had our normal workout. I then had a one-to-one session with one of my members, a short nap, and a 3-mile walk to the market and back. Not bad for a day after destroying a tumor in my brain! Modern medical technology is amazing!

THE GAME PLAN

It was *game on* for the main event: the elimination of lung cancer from my body. We all had a part to play: me, the doctors, and my support network. The doctors' job was to provide the right medicines and monitor our progress. My job was threefold: maintain a healthy mindset, eat the right foods, and exercise.

Everything I read about winning the cancer battle revolved around believing I was going to win and believing that nothing bad could befall me. Interestingly, I couldn't imagine being any other way. I knew I had what it would take to survive. I always believed that if someone else could accomplish something, then there was no reason I couldn't accomplish the same thing. I might have to work harder, study harder, ask for more help, or try new approaches, but other people beat this and so could I.

Nutrition and exercise are the keys to winning. Many cancer patients are done in by the chemo and their inability to function, to eat, and to take care of themselves while getting the treatment. I declared that day that I would not allow that to happen to me. I would eat even when I didn't want to; I would exercise even when I didn't want to, and I would continue to work and be an effective presence for my clients even when I didn't want to.

I would do all those things because I wanted to win. All my life I've had the ability to push through pain, and that experience was the precursor to my fight with lung cancer. I was ready for this.

I have always believed in the body's ability to heal itself. So, I called on my body to do its job. Through focus, meditation, conscious thought, alternative healing practices, and exercise I engaged my body in this battle.

A SECOND OPINION

The weekend after surgery, we went for a six-mile walk and golf on Saturday and a seven-mile walk and birthday party on Sunday. The great news is that the surgery worked faster than I anticipated; I was rapidly getting control back in my left hand. On Sunday, I went upstairs and started playing my ukulele. Teresa heard me and came up with tears in her eyes seeing me playing. What a joyful moment for both of us.

My playing wasn't good. I had about 90% control, but I could play songs!

"They didn't manage to improve your singing," Teresa teased.

For a second opinion, we met with the head of research at UCLA. He went over my files in detail. He had all the information in advance and was well prepared to discuss my case. He even had another doctor go over all the data with us before he got there.

Because I am a nonsmoker, he felt we needed to try for more genetic testing to determine if there were more targeted options for my treatment. He felt there were numerous opportunities and expected to find a targeted treatment that would work for us. It was great news as targeted treatment is not as harsh for the rest of the body. Again, they were talking about treatment designed to stop the growth, not necessarily designed to cure the cancer. UCLA would be sending their findings to my oncologist prior to our appointment. The doctor also suggested that we postpone the start of chemo. It would give me more time to recover from the brain surgery as well as giving us time to get the results of his additional tests.

Teresa and I discussed the idea of postponing chemo. We felt there would be no value in delaying the chemo and if a different strategy did present itself, we could always change course.

The doctor also said, "You may be an ideal candidate for a clinical study that I am leading with Novartis." We signed up for that as well. Kaiser sent my biopsy samples so that in a couple of weeks we would know if I qualified for the study. Bottom line: the second opinion was great! We felt much better informed and set to move forward.

TESTIMONIAL: MATT ERIKSON

I met Matt through Vistage. He was slated to be in a different Vistage group. But it turned out that there was a conflict of interest. He called me up while I was in Mexico and explained the situation. I told him of course I would make room in our group. Matt has become one of those friends that I'm not ashamed to say I love. Matt says:

> *"The first time we had lunch together, we went to the sushi place. I looked at the menu, and I thought about everything, trying to make my decision. It took me a while because I was reading all the descriptions and everything. So, I finally placed my order and then the waitress turned to Les."*
>
> *"Okay, how about you, sir?"*
>
> *Les said, "You guys make good sushi here, right?"*
>
> *She said, "Yes."*

He said, "So I'll take some of that. Send me out whatever is your favorite."

Two months after I was diagnosed with cancer, Matt found out that he had colon cancer. Instead of chemo, he had one surgery that removed the tumor. He counts his blessings. When asked about how I influenced him, he said. "I got lucky. It was scary, but it was also comforting to have someone to face it with. Les is so optimistic. His attitude is, 'If anybody's gonna knock this out, it's me.' I think the initial reaction is always, 'Why does this happen to good people?' I'm just pumped that he's been able to hang in there, inspire me and keep a positive attitude for the whole process."

LESSONS LEARNED: SCIENCE AND SPIRITUALITY

For years, I could never quite grasp why the worlds of science and spirituality were always at opposing ends when it came to viewing the vast awesomeness of the Universe; each arguing that they alone held the keys. Spirituality argues that science is too harsh and tangible, while from the scientific viewpoint, spirituality seems to be based on blind faith and guesswork. To me, it appears obvious that this limited perspective prevents *either* from having the keys, but also from even knowing which doors they open. Science and spirituality are stuck miles apart when they overlap in very elegant ways.

Enter *entanglement*, the incredible discovery of how two subatomic particles act like one object even when they are physically apart. If something happens to one of them, then instantaneously something happens to the other as if connected across space. But it doesn't stop there! Throughout the *entire* universe, particles and atoms act as if they are connected, suggesting that we are living within a holistic, deeply interconnected reality whose fabric includes the particles within our own bodies and minds. If that doesn't make you feel a little more significant than a speck on the universal tapestry, I don't know what will!

Mind-to-mind experiences have been reported throughout history by people of all cultures, ages, and educational backgrounds. This suggests that these phenomena are an integral part of the human experience. For centuries, the leading heads in science fought to disprove such experiences as mere coincidence or esoteric drivel. However, science itself, with the quantum theory of entanglement, gives us the proof of their measurable and tangible existence. Now the energetic connection between particles in our vast Universe, and in everything that resides in it, is the most logical explanation for these occurrences once considered supernatural. Well, that is just enough to make Buddha himself belt out "Eureka!"

It has always resonated deep within me that to fully grasp the magnificent Universe and its equally horrifying, beautiful expanse, you must be willing to view it from all angles. Furthermore, to observe what the physical world allows through the five senses, one must also use the observation techniques taught by Zen masters and yogis alike: transcendental viewing or *seeking with the soul* and *seeing with the heart*. In other words, you want to test hypotheses and run analyses, but also give equal feed to that inner voice and intuition. Both modes of exploring and learning from the world around me have always felt mutually important. And I can never look up at the stars without being equally as fascinated by the fact the twinkling I see is light-years away as I am with the feeling of connectedness that overcomes me.

Lung Cancer Fact Sheet | American Lung Association

> *"Though free to think and act, we are held together, like the stars in the firmament, with ties inseparable. These ties cannot be seen, but we can feel them."*
>
> **—Nikola Tesla**

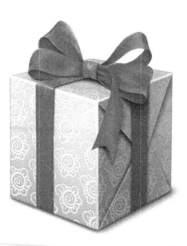

THE GIFT OF LEARNING

While learning about cancer was not my first choice, the knowledge required to remain the captain of my own ship (my body) was important to Teresa and me. We believed we could never have too much knowledge if we were going to persevere.

But, that's not the learning that truly matters.

I've always been a perpetual student (not a good one at first, but I found my stride). Learning about my clients, companies, customers, and friends has always been a foundational element of who I am; personally and professionally. In fact, my confidence of this attribute may have bordered on arrogance.

Cancer for the win.

I had no idea how *much* I would relish and lean into learning. Before cancer, I would certainly have deep dive conversations and analysis for my clients. Now, as my diagnosis has brought a heightened sense of clarity and presence, my thirst to learn has gone up.

In some cases, my curiosity may be as simple as something to do with the physics of a star as I gaze into the beautiful sunsets that blanket the Southern California coastline. Other times, as Teresa and I go for a long walk on a foggy morning, I would learn new things about her beliefs and thoughts that were never present in our "pre-cancer" conversations.

CHAPTER FOUR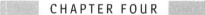

CHEMOTHERAPY

We met with the pulmonary oncologist and an hour later, found ourselves heading into our chemo orientation. We would learn the schedule for chemo among other things like how to prepare and what to expect.

I had been running out of steam every day since the brain procedure. I guess it took a greater toll on my body than I gave it credit for. Nothing an hour nap wouldn't cure, but it was a strange feeling for me to be low on energy. I expected to keep improving in the endurance arena, even during chemo. I was feeling ready and almost excited to see what my chemo would be like. I was expecting it to be tough but that I would handle it well.

Is that an odd thing to think?

I mean, who would seriously put the word "chemo" and "excited" in the same sentence?

If you've not figured it out by now, my belief systems have been naturally honed over the years to not always see the glass as half full. I have my share of moments where the reality can't be sugarcoated. It's deeper than that.

I do see the reality. However, when I separate my reality into facts vs. the present, something extraordinary occurs.

Being ready and excited for my first chemotherapy meant a new experience. OK, so it wouldn't be as cool as exploring a glacier, but bear with me...

Chemo may not look like fun, but in that moment of thought, I had not started. The actual chemo treatment was not for a few days. In the present moment, I felt fine. In that exact second, I did not experience *any* of the side effects of the treatment. Being present (and I mean 100% focused on that moment) naturally was not painful. My present condition plus the thought of my cancer going away or at least not ending my life early was the only thought that came to me.

In that moment, I was happy.

Still, it was a little surreal. Teresa and I were both experiencing moments where we looked at each other and just said, "Holy cow, we've got lung cancer and we are starting chemo!"

Our nephew, Ricky, had started chemo two weeks earlier. His lymph nodes were swollen all over his body. He was in a lot of pain and was struggling to keep his white blood cell count up. He lived alone in Las Vegas with very little support. I couldn't imagine going through the cancer treatment without Teresa, my friends, and the caring bridge community. I felt fortunate but also under an obligation to be there for Ricky as much as I/we could.

We bought him a gift card for Uber to make sure he could take care of his transportation needs. Teresa communicated with him daily while I remained on the periphery as I felt our common situation could be a little too real for Ricky.

I've always been active and a regular athlete. Routinely going to the gym not only made me physically strong, but the people and energy there reinforce a healthy environment. I was at the gym recently and a 50-year-old gentleman named Jason and I started a conversation. As we got to talking, Jason informed me that the doctors found a mass on his spine.

This guy was scared. I mean, he was frightened. I guess that's why he opened up to me. He didn't once talk about the fear of death. His 24/7 fear was for his family.

Jason had two kids in grade school and two in high school, minimal savings, and no life insurance. It wasn't as though he hadn't planned. As the founder of a small company, he considered his business his retirement vehicle. By the time his kids entered college, he planned to have things arranged with his business to not only afford University, but he would then sell his business to fund his retirement. He was just a few years away from execution on his plan when he got the cancer news.

"I quickly realized that my business would evaporate without me," he said. "My business was profitable, but only if I was steering the ship." His eyes drifted off as though he had just put it all on black at the roulette table. He had to rethink his entire personal and financial plan in a very short amount of time while simultaneously dealing with the fear of near term incapacity or death.

I might have been the only person he reached out to besides his family. I could only hope my mindset, words of encouragement and my friendship would help him as he discovered what lay ahead. It was sad that he felt he was not able to talk to other people.

What about you?

If you have cancer or have someone close to you with cancer, please find a way to connect and embrace human interaction. This is not a journey that should be suffered alone. Don't be afraid of doing or saying the wrong thing, your presence and willingness to engage will make a huge difference. It's rarely a fun conversation. Many people don't know what to say. I've had plenty of people who blurted out awkward ideas and even selfish quips.

However, no matter how one interacts, there is one underlying foundation that matters.

As long as you converse from a place of love, you cannot lose.

AFTERNOON CHEMO ORIENTATION

The doctor decided on a course of action. We were moving forward. We did not discount the next generation sequencing tests that UCLA prescribed. Kaiser did not offer that test, but they did have another one. I was pressuring my doctor to ask for it. If he failed to make it happen, I considered just doing the test through UCLA and paying for it myself. I was also still on the list for the clinical tests that UCLA was offering.

I would start chemo at 9:00 a.m. Friday. The first six sessions were going to be three doses of drugs: Pemetrexed, Carboplatin, and Keytruda. The next 35 sessions would be Pemetrexed and Keytruda and if I was still going strong, the next 100 sessions would be Keytruda only. The chemo treatments would be every three weeks on a Friday. I was told that they would take up to four hours to pour all this medicine (poison?) into my system. The three weeks between sessions would give my body time to feel like crap and then recover...if all went as planned.

Everything suddenly began to feel more real, more present, and scarier than it had before. I was in a state of low energy, feeling melancholy, and lost about what was in store for Teresa and me. While we knew what we were walking into, we had no idea how my body and my psyche would respond to the chemo. The "looking forward to" and odd "excitement" about the treatment was gone.

See? It's not all Pollyanna and rainbows.

The void of uncertainty allowed fear to seep in. I felt as if I was bouncing on an emotional trampoline.

I didn't like it. I couldn't stop it. My only choice was to embrace it. Fear is natural, after all. Our primitive brains' "fight or flight" response allowed us to evolve and thrive for millions of years. Trying to avoid or bury fear is temporary and fleeting.

I turned my thoughts not to the future, but to the past.

My past, like everyone else's, is peppered with challenges and triumphs. Every time my company increased in value, or a consulting client shared their success, my skills and strength increased. Going through hard times and coming out better off at the other end also increased my skills and strengthened me. Being able to overcome adversity became a shield that hardened further the more it was soaked in challenges.

I reflected on my shield.

Even though this new challenge was the most serious (life ending) possible, that never changed, not who I am, but who I have become. My journey, maybe like yours, molded my character.

Looking forward, we naturally look at the present circumstances and rarely into our character in that moment.

Looking back, I could see the event, but now, I could clearly see the molding of my character traits.

Over the years, I became stronger, and I never stopped believing in my strength. Overcoming personal, professional, and legal challenges expanded my ability to overcome adversity, and I never stopped believing in positive outcomes. All these journeys were one of learning, growth, and pain

Pain.

Oh, back to that word. I guess there would be more pain coming. Nobody looks forward to that, but if I weighed my character against potential pain, I believed character would win. That said, I had never been a chemo patient before. I was wondering if I could handle the discomfort and if my belief in who I am would win out. One thing was for sure: we would know soon. The fact that my doctor scheduled over five years of treatments as a minimum, told us we were in for the long haul. Teresa was of a similar state of mind. She just knew that she wanted to be right beside me throughout our journey.

We both felt a little lost as well.

The night before, I did not sleep well. I think I am uncomfortable with the unknown. Not knowing how I was going to react to the chemo was a little unsettling. My plan was to document chemo day as I went through it and then finalize a blog post that evening. It was weird to think that my new life protocol was going to be chemo treatment every third Friday for the foreseeable future. An added insult was that every medical professional frowned on us taking commercial flights. We had been planning on taking trips to Hawaii and the northwest. We would have to wait and see how my blood handled the chemo. If my white cells didn't go all wonky, maybe we could fly. It was another wait and see moment.

4:30 a.m.

I woke up and was at the gym by 5:00. Nothing earth shattering happened at the gym; it seemed like a normal workout. I went back home to have a protein shake before heading out for the oncology center. I got word from the doc that our next generation genetic sequencing tests had been ordered. That meant we were moving forward on two fronts. Those tests would take a couple of weeks.

9:00 a.m.

I was called in for my chemo treatment. A brightly lit beige room with nineteen cubicles for patients to get their chemo treatments waited for me. I was taken by the starkness and sterility of the room. There were no pictures on the walls or rugs on the floor, just a big reclining chair for me, a visitor's chair for Teresa, an IV stand, and a computer. I brought my ukulele to play during treatment, but the nurse put an IV in my hand, so that activity was out.

I was filled with anxiety about how my body would react. It was weird, I felt calm and tense at the same time. My nurse, Jesse, was upbeat and positive. He said that the three different medicines I am taking are not too bad for most people to handle. I liked hearing that. He also said that I was one of the fittest people he had seen and that was always good for minimizing the impact of the chemo.

> *"I never stopped believing in my strength, my ability to overcome adversity, and my ability to push through pain."*
>
> **—Les Whitney**

It was hard to believe how much had happened in the past two months. I had a vision board full of work accomplishments, personal growth, and travel. We cancelled trips to Anghor Wat and Vietnam, Hawaii, Holland for bicycling, and Iceland for the northern lights. I committed to transitioning from playing the ukulele to becoming a musician. Cancer hijacked my focus and turned it definitively toward my health. I decided that after my next chemo treatment on March 22, I would take some time to create a new vision board based on our new reality.

The old dreams were displaced. New dreams tried to break through the mortar of cancer.

11:30 a.m.
Chemo was complete. Three bags of medicine were weaving their way through my blood system. We were going after the cancer aggressively and it felt good to be on the offensive. I was completely whopped. It was more the emotional toll than the procedure, but it was still exhausting.

I needed a nap.

RECOVERY: SLEEP IS THE NAME OF THE GAME

My reaction to the chemo was better and different than I expected. From the moment we left the chemo ward, I was lethargic, surly, and foggy headed. We returned home about 1:00 p.m. on Friday and I just plopped myself down in front of the TV. I couldn't focus on reading and did not want to talk to anyone who called. I even barked at Teresa once. She's the love of my life, but she's not a pushover. In fact, Teresa has the nicest way saying the sweetest words wrapped inside a bacon sandwich of a threat.

"Why Les, not only am I your devoted wife, but I am also your caregiver. It would be a tragedy if I was only your wife."

Her devilish smile created in my mind visions of a nurse Ratched replacement. Or worse, Teresa stays, and I have to haul my sorry butt to the doctor's alone.

I smiled, nodded, and replied, "My love, you have 100% job security in all areas." She saw my previously snippy bark was replaced with a genuine smile that said, "I am sorry, please forgive me, it won't happen again."

I finally went to bed at 6:00 p.m. and slept right through until 6:00 a.m. Saturday morning. We went to the gym at 8:00 a.m. and I did an hour on the treadmill. After that, I returned home for another hour of sleep. I went back to my mindless watching the TV and found time for another two-hour nap. Sleep, sleep, sleep! Finally, I went to bed at 8:00 p.m. Saturday and awoke at 6:00 a.m. the next morning.

I felt amazing Sunday morning. There was no fogginess from too much sleep, no aches and pains from the chemo, no nausea, and no flu like symptoms, just normal relaxed Sunday morning Les. Could it be this easy? It was too soon to tell. Later that morning, we planned to go for a slow paced five-mile walk around the harbor below our house.

I wanted to keep active. No, I had to stay active.

I kept visualizing my upper right lung where my tumor resided. I pictured little Pac-Man like critters attacking the tumor and eating it a little at a time. I could almost feel the movement and breakdown of the mass. I felt like if I could focus on the area, it would help my body fight off the intruder. True or not, it gave me a feeling of control.

The mind has more power than we can possibly understand at healing the body. The placebo effect is a real thing. Don't get me wrong, I'm not suggesting I could "think away" my cancer. All I know is that when our minds are idle, sabotaging thoughts can creep in almost without realizing it. Better to intentionally put the good thoughts in there.

Pac-Man it is. Gobble. Gobble.

Oh yes, and that easy feeling was gone by 2:00 p.m. as I fell back into my post chemo zombie like state.

We were moving so fast with all the tests, doctors' appointments, second opinions, scans, MRIs, brain surgery, etc. that moving and doing and fighting and planning and fearing and hoping had all become my new norm. It was time to slow down and process. I had three-week periods of chemo and recovery, so after the first treatment, there was suddenly time to reflect. It felt a little weird to be taking my foot off the gas pedal. We found ourselves waiting, watching, monitoring, reacting, and repeating.

CHEMO IMPACT MONDAY AFTER CHEMO

I was simply trying to get my arms around how the chemo cycles were going to impact me going forward. I could say I was blessed that the impact had not been harsh the first time. In fact, it was rather mild. That said, I didn't like it! The first couple of days I was just tired and found sleep to be the perfect solution. The last two days I woke up with energy and excitement to start the day. I was able to do my full workout in the morning and conduct my meetings with my members right after.

I was fine until about 2:00 p.m., when things began to change. I started feeling nauseous, tired, and headachy, something akin to a low-grade flu. I tried to tough out the nauseousness but could only manage for an hour before breaking down and taking an anti-nauseous pill. Thank goodness they worked almost instantly.

The bottom line is that I was suffering minimal symptoms from the chemo: a little bleeding of the gums, no hair loss, and slight flu like symptoms. In lucid moments, I had to consider myself lucky. The most significant impact of the chemo was psychological. I felt like I lost my joyful perspective on life. I was trapped in a state of *blah*!

I felt weighted down by the knowledge that this was only the first of a series of three-week cycles that I would have to be dealing with for the rest of my life. I am a firm believer in my ability to choose how I react to different situations, and I worked hard to find the feelings, beliefs, activities, mindset, and interactions that would bring me the most joy. I didn't think that my mental state would be the thing I needed to control the most.

TUESDAY AFTER CHEMO

The biggest challenge I faced on Tuesday was my energy level. I slowly felt a little stronger and more energized as each day passed, but I could only claim about 80% of my normal energy levels. I did not take a nap Monday, the first no nap day since the treatment. I considered that as an improvement, though a small one.

I was eating nonstop for three days (most cancer patients have trouble eating). I heard that keeping my weight up was important to ease the stress and duress of chemo. Teresa did a great job of keeping healthy, fresh, and easy to nibble on items in the fridge and cupboard. I needed to eat the right foods, minimizing sugar as much as possible. Cancer thrives on sugar. In fact, one of the CAT scans included injecting me with a glucose solution. When I saw the scan, the two spots with cancer lit up like a Christmas tree while the rest of the scan showed nothing. The scan technician said that that was all the glucose being attracted by the cancer.

On Wednesday, I was excited to report no nausea for two days in a row. Was I past it? I was starting to think that the worst of the first chemo treatment was behind me. I would still have to be concerned about my white blood cell count, especially as it related to my immune system. I would do blood work the day before the next round of chemo just to make sure my immune system was handling everything ok. Doctors and friends both told me that the chemo impact was cumulative. Just because I weathered the first treatment didn't mean I wasn't in for a bigger fight in the future. It seemed that regardless of my personality and way of being, cancer would not allow positive thoughts to take hold for an extended period of time.

WHAT'S THE PLAN?
I returned from a weekend retreat with fifteen other Vistage Chairs at the Rancho Bernardo Inn in San Diego. I shared my time with people who have a gift for knowing the right

questions to ask to bring me the greatest clarity. And, in my situation, clarity was the one thing most lacking.

What do I mean by clarity? Answers to questions such as:

1. What would "a good life for the rest of my life" look like?
2. Does my definition of a good life change if I have only until the end of 2019? How about five more years? How about ten more years?
3. What would be the best use of my time going forward?
4. How could Teresa and I maximize our time together?
5. What beliefs were serving me well in my condition and what beliefs should I let go?

On top of being satisfied with the conference, I was feeling lucky with my recovery as well. Eight days after chemo I felt strong all day with no side effects from the chemo. I didn't lose a strand of hair. I was almost embarrassed at how well I handled the treatment.

Part of my challenge was planning around the unknown and the biggest unknown was how long I would live. The likely scenario was one year. It could be five years, or it could be ten years, but those estimates were speculative. We just didn't know, and would it matter regarding my decision-making? I couldn't answer the question about what would make a good life going forward if I didn't know how long I had.

I was looking at my situation as if I needed to know the answer to that question, but then I came to a realization. The clarity I got around this was to live my life as if I only had that year. I would do what was right for my health but also what was right for Teresa and me to live each day to the fullest. It wouldn't be about compromise, it was about choosing the best course for us and making those choices every day.

Teresa and I decided to sit and talk and to make those major life decisions based on the best way to maximize every day we had left together. In an earlier post, I wrote that "prolonging my life means living my life!"

It was time to define *living my life*.

My decision-making revolved around three possibilities and one fear. The possibilities were that while Teresa and I had seen most of the world, there were places we had not seen, and I wanted to make sure to find a way to see those places. Some of the places that came to mind were Angkor Wat, Petra, and Ephesus. Travel was always important to us, and we didn't think it was time to compromise.

I probably should not have thrown out that old vision board.

Another possibility was to use the time I had left to share my gratitude with those people who guided me and/or walked beside me on my journey through life. And the final possibility was to continue my work in a way that I could be an effective mentor and catalyst for change while still making time for my treatments.

Gratitude is one of those rare things that are, like a smile, free to give away, you have unlimited supply, and both people benefit. Being grateful for others would create a spark of gratitude towards the other people they knew. And equally important, I could be grateful for myself.

My only lingering bit of fear was that if I made too much space in my life for travel, treatment, and Teresa, what would happen when I ran out of travel, or the treatments slowed down? I certainly could not sit around watching TV all day. Being lazy and unproductive was as foreign to me as wearing a suit and tie. The lingering fear soon started to grow on its own. What was a fleeting annoyance developed into full-time dread. The foreboding was deep-seated, growing, and as real as you are sitting where you are right now reading this.

Thankfully, that was not my only fear.

The fear of not enough time, travel, or treatments was no match for over 60 years of another fear. This other fear was battle-tested. This fear would be no match for the fear of making too much space… of giving cancer too much of my time.

The fear of not having truly "lived" each day vibrantly.

Forward.

With drive.

Naturally, living in the present is a foundational element of my growth and character. Being in the "now" and actively listening and engaging with those around me at a very high level had become second nature to me. But the moment my imagination created "out of travel" or "too much idle time," I knew I was in uncharted territory. I had to revisit my past and remind myself that my current feelings were temporary and reality was the same as before.

By reaching back and knowing how I got there, my zest for living completely obliterated the temporary thoughts of scarcity.

Regardless of my strength, the challenges continued.

I am not alone with my fears. We all have them. My friends, Teresa, my clients. Even my doctor had fears. His was the fear of exposing me to other people while my immune system was compromised by the chemo. I needed to come up with a strategy that would keep me relatively safe while allowing me to travel and interact with other cultures. There was nothing stopping me from sharing my gratitude with those who had helped me throughout my life except that I didn't want anyone to think that by sharing my gratitude, I was giving up on my future.

As the stoics professed, "The obstacle is the way." Teresa and I weaved a plan to maximize our travel while being mindful of my decreased immunity. It would be a balancing act that we closely monitored and were 100% truthful with how we felt.

I had already found that my clients were more than willing to be flexible around my time and my travel. Thank God for technology like Skype, FaceTime, and Zoom that allowed me to video conference from anywhere at any time.

I found it alarming that the biggest challenge in *living a good life for the rest of my life* was the vision of myself as a lazy person. I imagined that I had to fight every day to overcome that laziness. This self-talk likely came from some event in childhood and probably served me well through my school years and early career.

I think I've proven that this story is untrue, but it still lives inside of me. Yes, the fear survives. I was challenged by the belief that I would simply sit on my butt if I didn't have a plate full of things I "had to do." There was nothing in my recent history or behavior that would make me, or anyone believe this is true. I needed to confront the belief and make the space in my life if I was going to have the time and flexibility to live the life I wanted in the years ahead.

I led two group meetings last week and had several fabulous conversations each day. One topic that came up both days was effective use of our time. As one person said, "we spend so much of our energy building our financial bank, but what do we do to manage our time bank since we cannot give ourselves more time?"

- What are we doing that is more of a time eater than a value-add to the quality of our lives?
- If we were to treat our time as a limited resource, what would we do differently?
- What activities would we do more of and what would we stop doing?

From this conversation, I challenged myself and my members to not only create a "to-do" list, but to create a "not do" or "stop doing" list.

- What are those things that we can delegate or pay others to do?
- What are those things that drain our energy?
- And what are those things that use a lot of time for minimal value and keep us from other things of greater value?

The bottom line for Teresa and I was simple. We would hoard our time and choose to use our time on activities that brought us the maximum value and joy. Historically, I have said yes to most requests if I found the white space on my calendar. For some reason, I've looked at open time on my calendar as uncommitted time. I, therefore, said "yes" to whatever was asked of me even though I could use that time on more valuable and/or more enjoyable activities if I just stopped to think and said "no."

I committed to saying "no" more often.

Vistage speaker, Bruce Brier, talks about blocking out a couple of hours each day to devote to completing high priority work. He calls it PWT (priority work time). I intended to block several hours each day and mark it PT (priority time) and fill it with activities I enjoyed. Perhaps it would be priority work time, perhaps priority health time, and as often as possible, priority Teresa time.

I'm reminded of a stance I took with my employees when I was leading companies. I did not allow them to say "I did not have time" when they missed a commitment. They had to say, "it wasn't a priority." This made them think hard about where and on what they spent their time. This stance resonates strongly with me today in how I chose to spend my time.

I expected to continue feeling strong and healthy. I had a blood test on Thursday to make sure I was handling the chemo and my second chemo treatment on Friday morning. I was feeling blessed to have handled the chemo so well, I prayed that it continued to be something doable and not overwhelming. I was told that weight is my friend during chemo, so I was eating like a horse. Unfortunately, I gained four pounds with all that eating. I would have to decide if I should control my eating or buy new clothes.

SECOND ROUND OF CHEMO

I went to Kaiser to get my blood drawn and by the time I got home, the results were posted on my web portal. White blood cell count was good, red and platelets were a little low but not bad. Low red and platelets are a sign of anemia which could be why I spent so much time napping.

I approached my first chemo session with a great deal of apprehension and anxiety. Now that that 1st one (with 100% uncertainty on what would happen) was over, I was excited to experience the second one. I did so well on the first treatment, I was expecting and hoping to have a similar experience. If everything went as expected, I would have a much better understanding for how to schedule my life. For the time being, I kept my calendar wide open on Monday and Tuesday after chemo, expecting to have some difficulty recovering. I considered going down and spending the weekend at our home in Mexico. It would give me a chance to relax, sleep, and do very little after treatment.

One of my CEO groups arranged for meals to be delivered to us every week which simplified Teresa's effort. I received blankets for my chemo treatments, lots of books, and even nausea relief medicine.

I had an appointment with my oncologist on April 9, but we didn't plan to do any more CAT scans until after the 4th treatment (six more weeks). I didn't know what we would discuss on the 9th (perhaps the results of the genetic testing), but I did know that we wouldn't be able to tell how well the chemo was working that soon after treatment began.

I also had an appointment with the brain surgeon on April 19 to review the results of my stereotactic surgery. I had an MRI on my brain scheduled for April 9 as well. My hand was shaking again so I was anxious to see the results of the MRI and discuss how I was doing with the doctor.

I thought the first round of chemo might be too good to be true and it turned out that I was right. After my second chemo infusion Friday morning, everything seemed to be going well. I was not as drowsy as the first time, but my stomach was a little queasy. All said, things seemed about the same as the first chemo session.

Then Saturday came...

I drove us down to Mexico early Saturday morning. By the time we arrived, I was whopped. I spent 90% of my time Saturday in a horizontal position. I had flu like symptoms, queasy stomach, no energy, and it felt like I spent the entire day fading into and out of sleep. The expression, "felt like I got hit by a truck" was mild.

I got hit by a convoy of trucks.

My mind wasn't clear. I would try to read a bit. After a minute, I realized my eyes moved, but no words came into my brain. I tried writing. Within the first sentence, it was as if I didn't know what the point was. All cognitive endeavors were out of the question.

The convoy had apparently crushed my head so hard, my brain popped out like a grape. I was confined physically and intellectually. Even watching TV (when my eyes opened) was useless. The fog was dense and uncomfortable.

My gratitude for sleep increased.

Sunday was a little better. After eleven hours of sleep, we headed across the street to a great French breakfast place. My stomach was queasy again that morning, but other than that I felt great. I went on a four-mile walk later that day and everything seemed good until Monday when we decided to drive home.

As soon as we arrived at home, I knew something wasn't right. My stomach was in my throat, I had trouble sitting up without feeling sick and I couldn't focus. I ended up lying down in front of the TV doing whatever I could to feel comfortable. Nothing worked; I ended up going to bed at 8:00 p.m. Monday night and woke up at 8:00 a.m. Tuesday morning. I was up for an hour and then went back to bed at 9:00 a.m. waking again at 1:00 p.m. That time I stayed awake an hour and a half and went back to bed at 2:30 p.m. I woke up again at 5:00 p.m. and decided to try to eat something and to post an update. Unfortunately, there wasn't much to post.

I thought I was going to be a fortunate person with minimal side effects from the chemo.

No such luck.

The second round of therapy had other plans. All I could hope for was that the number of bad days would be minimal compared to the good days. This couldn't last forever.

Another person in my life was diagnosed with cancer; this time it was colon cancer. He was the fourth person close to me to be diagnosed since I got my news. He was a young man who recently started a new job, his wife was due with their first baby, and he was diagnosed with cancer. They were planning to take a chunk of his colon out the next week. I was determined to do all I could to be there for him.

If I thought I was too young for this, all these younger people were proving how terrifying this disease was. There was no fairness to it. There was no right person, no right time of life to be struck down. It was just an ugly disease that could take anyone it wanted to.

FEELING BETTER

Wednesday was a much better day and Thursday was even better! Cancer still sucks. Chemo still sucks. But I was beginning to think that if I only had four bad days out of every three weeks, I could live with that. I was working mornings when I had energy and then I would go home to nap. That seemed to be the correct recipe for me.

When we went to our appointments, we had a co-pay of $20. Kaiser didn't bill me one time and we received a note asking for payment. Teresa went into our portal to see what was going on and how to pay. What she discovered was all the accounting for my treatment.

Unless you are very close to the medical billing industry, you would not believe what chemo costs. At each session I got three different kinds of chemo; one cost $27,000, one cost $20,000, and the other cost $2,500. Coupled with the fees for nursing and room usage, it cost about $55,000 every time. If I was going to get chemo every three weeks for a year, my treatment would cost about $935,000. If we added up all the doctor fees, PET Scans, MRIs, and additional costs, I could quickly see cancer was not a cheap thing.

One million dollars a year.

It took me a long time to adjust to feeling sick all the time. Historically, I plowed through sickness and injuries as if they did not exist. My body and mind had not yet figured out how to plow through cancer so I had to learn to slow down, to take what I could from each day, and to rest when I needed to rest. It was harder on me mentally than physically because I kept judging myself, expecting to be tougher and stronger. I was getting lots of good advice to go with the flow, to rest, to allow my body to dictate my needs but still it was hard to follow.

One significant challenge was that the chemo caused short-term havoc on my red blood cells. By the weekend (day 8 after chemo), I felt 100%. In fact, my endurance after more than a week was as good as it had been since before we worked on the brain tumor five weeks prior.

I felt "strong like ox!"

On Friday, I received a package from a local middle school. Apparently, my friend's son attended this middle school and shared my story with his classmates. The students each sat down and wrote me sweet personal notes of encouragement. As I read each note, I couldn't stop the tears from rolling down my cheeks and blurring my eyes. It was amazing how impactful a simple note could be. I was reminded that I could be sending more notes of encouragement and appreciation as well.

THIRD, FOURTH, & FIFTH TREATMENTS

One thing about the chemo process is that there is no shortage of time between sessions. I was doing great over the two healthy weeks, living my life like a normal, cancer-free human being. I felt as healthy as I have ever been. The only symptom I was experiencing was a mild case of "chemo belly" which is a low-grade sourness in the stomach that just lingers. It wasn't anything debilitating, just a nuisance. I imagined that people who saw me might think, "what is the hubbub over this cancer stuff? Les looks and acts as healthy as ever." It was difficult to reconcile the shortened lifespan with feeling strong and healthy.

I did have my moments. One evening, Teresa and I watched a sad film and I just started crying. Soon, Teresa's tears had joined mine and we sat and cried and talked about our fears of losing time together, of the suddenness of my diagnosis, and the frustrations of all the unknowns. This was the third time that we cried since the diagnosis, and I was confident that it wouldn't be the last.

> *There was no fairness to it.*
> *There was no right person, no right time*
> *of life to be struck down. It was just an*
> *ugly disease that could take anyone*
> *it wanted to.*

I decided to fit in as much travel as possible during the last eight months of my first cancer year and on into the future. The operative word is "fit in." The chemo process knocked six days out of every three-week period. On Thursdays, I had my pre-chemo blood test, Friday was chemo day, and then from Saturday until Tuesday I just felt awful. That left me with fifteen healthy days to enjoy in each cycle.

The problem was that I had group meetings on the second Wednesday and Thursday of each month, and I needed to reserve time to facilitate twenty, hour and a half to two-hour one-to-one meetings each month. It became hard to find a consecutive seven days to travel. I scheduled three five-day trips, so that was a win. I was determined to make time for a trip to Hawaii and a trip to Europe, but I couldn't figure out when. Some of the decision process depended on the effectiveness of the chemo.

After so many treatments, I became anxious to know if it was doing its job:

- Was my tumor shrinking?
- Had my tumor simply stopped growing?
- Was the tumor *still* growing?
- Did I have new tumors throughout my body?

All of these were possible, and the answers would dictate how Teresa and I proceeded with both health and life decisions. At this point, I was still awaiting the results of the genetic testing. I was so hopeful that I fit the criteria for targeted therapy which is more effective and less invasive. My gut told me what I already knew, but I tried to remain hopeful.

My left hand still did not have enough control to play the ukulele well which was frustrating. I wouldn't know the results of the brain MRI until I met with the surgeon on April 19th. There was so much damn waiting. There were so many damn unknowns.

While I had hoped things would be different, my oncologist confirmed that I would be getting chemo every three weeks for the rest of my life since my cancer was deemed "incurable." But he also said that the most destructive of the three types of medicines would be dropped after the fourth to sixth chemo session. I hoped that change would lessen the impact the drugs were having on my system and perhaps shorten the recovery time.

Disappointing news from the doctor revolved around my cell samples for the genetic testing. Neither UCLA nor Kaiser said there were enough cell samples to test my cancer for the right genetic markers for targeted therapy.

"Just get more samples," you might say.

Unfortunately, when they did the procedure to get the original sample, the surgeon said he did the best he could do to get the limited cells he got. They would have to do a more invasive procedure to get more samples. The effectiveness of that procedure wasn't guaranteed since hopefully the lung tumor had already shrunk, and there would be less of a sample to go after. The decision was to do a new CT scan in four months to see *how much* the tumor shrunk and then decide whether to try for another sample or not.

We also planned another MRI on my brain. I was getting used to these MRIs because I fell asleep during the last procedure. Obviously, I was not as stressed out by the MRI as I was the first time. It was a little victory but would take them where I could find them.

I felt occasionally as if nothing was going on with me and this was all a dream. How could I possibly have cancer if I felt and looked like I did? If it wasn't for the pictures of the tumor and the immediacy of the treatment, I might think it was all a hoax.

Special note: Teresa demanded a name change from "Chemo Fridays" to "Healing Fridays!" It's all in the mindset! From then on, that's what we called it.

Healing Friday. Has a nice ring to it, doesn't it?

The next "Healing Friday," I felt strong and unaffected. Same thing Saturday when I walked six miles to meet Teresa at her garden sale. Sunday, I started to slow down a bit and by Sunday night I could hardly function. I slept eleven hours and woke up with the worst case of chemo belly ever. I didn't feel like eating, didn't feel like talking, didn't feel like reading, I just wanted to go back to sleep.

As usual with me, I did see a shining light ahead. With a few rounds of chemo behind me, I could be sure that by Wednesday I would be feeling better. Add to that the fact that the plan was to cut back from three bags of chemo to two, eliminating the nastiest, most debilitating of the medicines. I wouldn't let the disease keep me down!

Logistically speaking, I had some work to do over the next month. I discovered that I was facilitating a weekend retreat starting the afternoon of my next chemo treatment. I just couldn't imagine how that would be possible. I decided to reach out to my colleagues to see if one or two of them could help. I also asked a few of the participants to lead sections of the meeting. I would be there for support, but I took the mantle of responsibility off my shoulders.

The Orange County Chair community stepped up to help me out with the retreat. I would just need to coordinate with the chairs and throw an agenda together. I also had numerous texts and voice messages to return. Even cancer couldn't empty my inbox!

To ease my burden going forward, my Vistage members committed to scheduling their one-to-one time with me for the rest of the year. This would be instead of scheduling each meeting as it came or only a few weeks out. The hope was that knowing what was on my plate ahead of time would give me a better idea of how to work around treatments and hopefully travel. The only challenge was that the schedule itself would be a chore and I didn't have the energy for it right away.

One time after treatment, I spent almost sixty hours in bed with no desire to communicate with anyone. It took me that long to climb back to my normal self. They said at the beginning that chemo was cumulative; each session being a little tougher through the first four or five sessions and they were right! All energy and strength was zapped from my body. And so much for the "no weight loss" attempt. I dropped from 173 to 166 in just a week.

Time for a confession. The only time I felt halfway decent during chemo is when I took THC at night. The THC allowed me to lay flat, relax, and glide off into sleep. Teresa thought that since I was not functioning coherently anyway, I should take THC first thing when I wake up and stay under the influence throughout the five days of chemo and its recovery. I didn't really enjoy the buzzed feeling, but it did sound like a good alternative to misery.

When we finally visited the brain surgeon to review the MRI, we waited in the room the nurse had directed us to, filled with both hope and apprehension. Did they get it all? Were there any new masses that developed in the past month? The room was thick with tension, but I was calm and prepared for whatever the doctor would say. The real concern was the result of the CT scan; would it tell us that the chemo was working, would it tell us the mass in my lung was stable or shrinking, or would it tell us the chemo wasn't working and the mass had grown and there were new masses in other parts of my body?

When the doctor walked in, there was a hop in his step and a huge smile on his face. First, he said, "you appear to be handling the chemo better than most and you appear to be getting great results!"

That alone was great news without any specifics. Then he said, "The MRI shows that we got all of the cancer in the brain. Further, your swelling is gone, and your brain is healing better and faster than expected." As far as the brain tumor was concerned, his work was done, and he did not expect to have any new brain work on me in the near future.

He then said, "I've looked at the CT scan and while that is not my expertise it is apparent that the lung cancer is at worst static and at best shrinking." There was no cancer anywhere else in my body so they hoped it was arrested. All in all, the doctor seemed quite optimistic that we would be visiting them at Kaiser for a long while.

What did it mean?

First, I would continue the chemo treatment indefinitely into the future. I was already tired of chemo and didn't realize how beat up and defeated I was by the treatments and by not knowing whether they were working or a waste of time. Once I knew it was working, my tolerance increased markedly.

The doctor also said that they did not want to do anything about the cancer in my lungs because it had already entered my blood. He believed we could, and perhaps should, go in with radiation therapy and destroy the lung cancer. He thought that the chemo had the circulating cancer somewhat under control so we might as well get rid of the other tumor. The plan was to wait until the end of July to verify that everything was under control and if it was, go in and kick the lung cancer butt's cells.

When the brain doctor walked out of the room, Teresa and I looked at each other, reached over and hugged and started crying. We held in so much emotion throughout the process, and with the first indication from a doctor that things were going well, we just burst into tears. I had not realized that I was operating on a 12-month timeline and wondering if the chemo was worth it. I was better prepared to fight going forward knowing that we might be enjoying chemo for many, many years.

We still had a long battle ahead. We had not spoken to our primary oncologist yet. However, this little piece of good news had us invigorated and ready to fight on. Teresa and I booked a trip to Sedona, a trip to Monterrey/Pebble Beach, a trip to Hawaii, and a bike and barge in Holland. I was back on the travel circuit. It felt so good to have something to look forward to besides meeting with my clients and counting the days to my next chemo treatment. I still couldn't imagine making big decisions about life like moving or retiring, but decisions that affect the next two years were open game. It felt so good to think about other things besides cancer!

TESTIMONIAL: DAVID SPANN

David is a Vistage chair I took under my wing, when I was busy establishing chairs and helping new groups evolve. When you give value to other people, you always receive something in return. I got a friendship that has become an important source of strength in my life. David got help establishing his Vistage group, and we were both able to broaden our community. In that way, it truly is better to give than it is to receive.

David says:

The first time I met Les would have been April 2010. I was just starting out as a Vistage chair. Down in San Diego, there is an introductory training process, and back then it was eight days of heavy bombardment with information. "Here's how all this is going to work, here's what you do," that sort of thing. Les was one of the trainers and something really clicked. I felt like he knew what he was talking about and could help me through the process. We were each supposed to have a Market Mentor. I was the only one from Boise, so there was no Market Mentor in my area. That meant somebody from outside of my market was going to have to help me. I just decided, "You know what? I'm going to ask Les."

He said, "Well, I think they've already got somebody for you."

I said, "I'm sure they do. But I don't know who that is. And I know you. So, I'm asking you, would you be willing to do it?"

He said, "Heck, yeah!"

So, we began our relationship as two folks who were willing to step outside of the norm.

LESSONS LEARNED: CHEMO SUCKS!

Chemo got its start after World War II when doctors discovered that service men who were exposed to mustard gas developed toxic changes in bone marrow cells. Further research indicated that nitrogen mustard was an effective treatment against lymphoma. Not only does it feel like poison, but it literally is poison. The same medicine used in chemotherapy was originally designed to hurt people.

In 1956, methotrexate was first used to "cure" cancer.[1] Although some cancer, like mine, is incurable, we still use chemotherapy to control it and alleviate the symptoms.

Throughout this book, I have made many references to how difficult and upsetting chemo is. From the strange recovery pattern to the plethora of side effects, it isn't something I would wish on my worst enemy. I don't need to repeat myself, but I'll say it again.

CHEMO SUCKS!

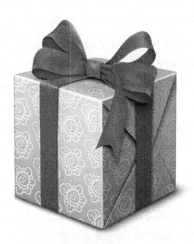

THE GIFT OF GRATITUDE

This chapter of the book has more "play by play" than reflection and ideas.

And that was on purpose. As you know, I started a blog at CaringBridge.org to document my journey. I started this with no specific intention beyond sharing the chaotic,

---

1   History of Cancer Treatments: Chemotherapy

emotional path that follows a cancer diagnosis. At the time, getting a cancer diagnosis put me into a new fraternity.

But, documenting this journey has benefited not only my many friends and associates, it has benefited many people I have never met in person. For that I am extremely grateful!

Which brings me to the gift of gratitude. There is no way I could express enough the gratitude I feel for all who have followed me and supported me on this journey. By sharing how grateful I am, I ensure that they know they've made a difference and hopefully will continue to make a difference for others in the future.

Because so many have expressed their gratitude to me for my blog and my openness, I've decided to seek a larger audience via this book. Their gratitude has inspired me to give more, to share more, and to write more.

Gratitude is like a flywheel. The more we share our gratitude, the more of what we are grateful for we receive. The more one receives expressions of gratitude, the more they are inclined to repeat the behavior. Gratitude is the gift that keeps on giving.

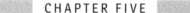 CHAPTER FIVE

THE NEW NORMAL

While I was not looking forward to the four days after chemo, I was excited to be getting chemo since my past results had been so good. Our lives had changed so much in the past few months. The three-week chemo cycle had become my new normal, so adjusting our living patterns to the cycle was important and valuable. I could be a little bit whiny and a bit of a baby during those chemo days, but our lives quickly reverted to the new normal soon after treatment. I still worked, we exercised every day, found ways to eat nourishing meals even when I didn't feel like eating, and we had plenty of time for friends, family, and fun. I even became comfortable with my frequent naps.

During this journey, it became quite clear that many people have an enormous fear of cancer, even if they don't have it. As soon as I mentioned the word, people would either try to change the subject, their eyes would well up with tears, or they didn't know what to say. I had four friends and family who were diagnosed with cancer in the four months since my diagnosis. The initial fear they all expressed was a little scary for me.

While I had my share of anxious moments, overall, I can't say a feeling of fear was prevalent. I kept wondering, *what is wrong with me that I have not had any fear?* The more I learned, the more I realized that fear wells up at different stages of the journey. There is no common bell curve, mind you. Each person's fear comes and goes depending on a host of circumstances. One person's fear may be greater at the onset and another one may fear the side effects of treatment. I am stunned and encouraged by the number of people I meet who have been through some type of cancer treatment and are now on the other side. Many say they are in remission. "Remission" does not mean cancer free; it simply means it is controlled all the way up until it isn't any longer. Remission can last 6 months or 60 years.

DEATH!?!

Most people seem to be uncomfortable talking about death and dying. Regardless of how well my treatment was going, I still have an elevated risk of dying in the very near future. Although my timeline improved markedly with the success of my treatments, mind you.

But the risk remains.

We are all going to die someday. My final days just have the strong possibility of being sooner than any of us want. What I found interesting was how upset my friends and colleagues got when I talked openly about death. It seemed that talking about it made it too real for some. For me, it was simply the reality of my journey. I was living every day in the moment! The prospect of death was of near-term concern to me. I am not necessarily stoic. For me, death is probably like it was before I was born.

Nothing.

My condition allowed me to talk openly about my situation. As it turns out, the "gifts" of cancer became existing things we all know and often take for granted. While I sum these up at the end of each chapter to satisfy our linear brains, in truth, they are all intertwined.

Journaling, speaking, and even embracing that cancer accelerated the date of my demise has focused my thoughts and energies in many ways, encouraging me to:

- Live every day fully, vibrantly, and fully aware of everything.
- Take nothing for granted and express that gratitude silently or openly.
- Love my friends, family, and Teresa more passionately.

Every day is a gift to be experienced to the fullest. I was always focused on making a difference in the lives of everyone I met. My cancer laser focused these encounters to a new and very satisfying level. Even as I write this, I enjoy every experience. I love being present and compassionate with others.

And loving Teresa well beyond her expectations has never been easier.

Cancer gave me the opportunity to see the world through new eyes; to enjoy the colors of all the flowers, the smells in nature, the joy in spending time with others, and even the joy in feeling better on Wednesday after chemo.

THE RETREAT

Karen Baez, Michele Jewett, and Sherri Nooravi stepped up to help with my retreat. Karen would lead my group on Friday and try out her new Vistage presentation. Michele would drive down to La Jolla on Saturday morning and run the meeting Saturday with Sherri stepping in to speak. And then there was Jes Liu, one of my members, who took complete control of all the planning and logistics for the retreat. What was looking like a stressful, challenging weekend would suddenly be a relaxing chemo filled weekend.

I had my infusion on Friday morning, then jumped into the car to the weekend retreat in San Diego. We didn't get fifteen miles before I had to pull over and let Teresa drive. As soon as Teresa took over, I was out like a light.

I was scheduled to kick off the meeting at noon with my members. When my part was done, I unceremoniously laid down on the floor and fell asleep as they continued the meeting. I suspect they were able to ignore my snoring!

We had a nice dinner planned for Friday evening, but I wasn't feeling up to it. I passed out and went back to sleep from 6:00 p.m. until 5:00 a.m. As usual, chemo days one and two were all about sleep.

Saturday morning, we met with the group for breakfast and another speaker. As soon as the speaker started, I was back on the floor sleeping (yes, and snoring again). I played nine holes of golf before Teresa dragged me back to the room to rest up for our group dinner.

I was exhausted.

Monday morning, we woke up to the alarm at 4:15 a.m. and headed to the gym. After 40 minutes of light cardio, I called it quits and we headed for home. As soon as we arrived at the house, I marched upstairs and jumped into bed for another five hours of sleep. I couldn't get out of bed after that. My body ached all over, chemo belly was raging, and my head was in a fog. This continued through Tuesday. I finally got out of my pajamas and into my work clothes Wednesday morning. I know I've mentioned this before, but chemo really sucks.

This time around, the cycle of abuse made it hard for me to maintain a positive attitude. I kept picturing going through it every three weeks for the rest of my life. Thinking of the futility of recovery each time brought up nothing but dread. The good news was that once I had a good day the tough days didn't look so bad. I was heartened by the thought that we would be cutting back on the nastiest of the chemo during the next session. I could only hope that I was not putting too much stock into the cutback. I really didn't want to be disappointed and have an equally awful experience the next time around. It was the first time in my life that I wasn't looking forward to the future.

> *Cancer gave me the opportunity to see the world through new eyes; to enjoy the colors of all the flowers, the smells in nature, the joy in spending time with others.*

Cancer has definitely changed my perspective on life.

I was always a "what's next?" kind of person. I looked forward to the next opportunity, adventure, person to know, tidbit to learn, or challenge to take on. Now, the future has become more about how to survive and how to enjoy what was available. The anticipated future was limited to the next few months rather than the next few years.

I completely shifted how I found joy!

I found myself much more appreciative of every interaction and experience, I found joy in almost every conversation, and I cherished my relationships. That was a good outcome of cancer. The bad outcomes may seem obvious, but I found myself ranking them in order of their importance. The loss of hope for an active, adventure filled future was one of the worst. I had to adjust my dreams into two-week increments around the chemo.

Who was I to complain? One of my Vistage members, Nathaniel, has a 1 1/2-year-old daughter who was born with a tumor in her foot. A few weeks prior, they decided to amputate the foot. A biopsy of the tumor revealed malignant cancer. Beautiful Jubilee was recovering from and adjusting to losing her foot, which would be hard enough on anyone, let alone an infant and her parents. Now, in addition to prosthetics, they had to start her on chemo treatments. The good news was that her type of cancer had an 85% to 90% survival rate. I couldn't imagine a toddler like Jubilee going through everything I was going through. At least I could understand what was going on and why it was happening. For her, it was simply pain and misery.

A note about Jubilee. As I am writing this book, Jubilee is running around like a normal four-year-old except she has a hitch in her get-along from the prosthetic leg. She appears completely unfazed by her experience. She has even pulled off the prosthetic and shown it to curious children she meets on the playground. I am inspired by her and in awe of her ability to move forward in life as if nothing has happened.

CAREGIVERS

I was following Jubilee's CaringBridge site, and it reminded me of the pain, sorrow, love, hope, despair, and helplessness that our caregivers must feel every moment they are dealing with our cancer. Teresa was so diligent, so caring, so thoughtful, and so giving! I was getting the feeling that everyone who found themselves in the "caregiver" position had to give up a lot to create the time to be a great caregiver. At least in Teresa's situation, she could talk to me about my needs. She could express her love and get love in return. We could talk about the future and share our hopes for a silver lining on the other side.

Jubilee's mother, Brianna, had it even tougher. Jubilee didn't understand why she was being put through the wringer. Brianna had to stay strong in her presence, had to be mother, nurse, nurturer, disciplinarian, and chauffeur (among so much more). We were fortunate that I had already lived a long full life.

Teresa and I could rejoice in what we had.

If you have people in your life who have been thrust into the caregiving role, please be patient and understanding with them. Give them as much of your love and attention as you give to the patient in their lives. They need to know that they are supported. They need your words of love and encouragement. They don't need you to ask how they are doing, just assume that things are challenging and be present to whatever needs (expressed or unexpressed) they might have.

I didn't know how to make the situation easier for Teresa. It tore her up when I struggled with the chemo, and there was nothing I could do to ease her concern. I knew that her life was upended by my cancer, and she had become dependent on my attitude, the doctor's skills, and the power of the treatments. In a way, she was so powerful but also powerless. I needed her and yet where it counted, there was little she could do.

It was very disheartening and the ultimate smack in the face. How could I lean on her 24/7 when I knew I wouldn't be there for her to lean on?

CHEMO CUTBACK IS CONFIRMED

We met with the oncologist and made decisions about what to do moving forward. First, we would drop the more poisonous of the chemo effective that Friday. The chemo we would drop was carboplatin. This drug, while effective in killing the cancer, is also effective at killing the kidneys. I would continue with Keytruda (immunotherapy) and pemetrexed (chemotherapy).

My oncologist was not keen on radiation for the lungs. He said it might be too much for my body to handle. He planned to discuss his concerns with the radiation oncologist and would get back to me. We would make the final decision later.

The *great* news was that the lung cancer was smaller. The oncologist said that the scan results, while positive, might even be better than they seemed because the CT scan could not differentiate between live cancer cells and scar tissue. He said that the cancer likely shrunk more than the scan shows. We would know more when we completed both an MRI on my brain and the PET scan on the rest of my body another few months down the road. The PET scan would show more of the cell activity, how much of it is destroyed, and if there was any new activity.

Three days into the new chemo program, and not much had changed in how I responded to the medicine. I was tired and lacked all ambition: didn't feel like talking, writing, working, or pretty much anything. I did take my usual five-mile walk both on Saturday and Sunday so at least I could say that I was remaining active. I felt great on Monday and was hoping that would signal the end of the five-day recovery periods.

One of the CEOs I mentor mentioned to me that he was embarrassed to say my cancer had become a blessing in some ways. He, and many others, have said they are much more appreciative of their families and loved ones because of my journey. I've had several people tell me they are much more conscious of how they use their time, the choices they make, and how they determine what is important in every moment. I've had numerous conversations with people who have been working to get their affairs in order should they become ill or incapacitated because of my sudden, surprising diagnosis. Most importantly, the level of love, appreciation for others and life in general, and the awareness that we can do good in the world regardless of our circumstances increased dramatically.

Sometimes I felt like a fraud with this cancer. I looked the same, I acted the same, and if you saw me on the streets, you would never assume I was fighting cancer. My oncology nurse said that my symptoms were among the mildest she has seen. So, while I complained about the chemo, my reaction to cancer and chemo was much better than most cancer patients. I felt a little guilty too, because so many other people had it worse. Perhaps it was the result of a healthy lifestyle, and I should appreciate that.

The bottom line was, *I WAS BLESSED!*

Reducing my chemo intake by one bag did not have the effect I had hoped for. The severity of the chemo on my body and mind was not as extreme as it once was, but it was still significant. Sadly, the recovery seemed to linger longer, well into Wednesday. I scheduled four one-to-one meetings on Wednesday (each meeting would take about 2 hours and I had to drive between them) so I was very tired by the end of the day.

We drove down to Mexico where two very exciting things happened! First, I paddled out and surfed for the first time since I was diagnosed. I surfed like a 64-year-old man but at least I surfed. It felt good to be out there with my buddy Craig catching waves and chatting with the other surfers in the water. There was a normalcy out there that I was trying to create in all areas of my life. It felt good! I was determined to try a morning surf, eighteen holes of golf, and perhaps a four-mile walk. That historically has been my typical day in Mexico.

The second exciting thing that happened was that I was able to sit in my chair overlooking the ocean and play my ukulele for at least an hour. It was the first time Craig and I had played since I discovered my left hand no longer functioned in December. It was as if everything in my life was heading back towards normal. Craig brought his guitar down and I brought my amplifier and we played all night. I was concerned that surfing and ukulele would no longer have a place in my life. I was glad to put those concerns behind me.

IT'S HEALING FRIDAY AGAIN

We woke up at our normal time, went to gym, and returned home for breakfast just like any other day. We then packed up our supplies (food, water, and reading materials) and a gift for the chemo nurses. Teresa was very creative with her gifts each time. What she brought that day was not for the nurses. Teresa had crocheted about 10 beanie hats in bright colors to be given to chemo patients who had lost their hair. I was confident they would be appreciated.

Upon arriving at the chemo center, Randy (the check-in lead) greeted us with a "Hello Mr. and Mrs. Whitney," cheering us up and confirming that we came there way too often. We entered the 4th floor chemo ward which was filled with bald patients and their dedicated caregivers. It was surprising how jovial and upbeat several of the patients were! They brought a smile to my face. Once called in for treatment, they assigned me to one of nineteen alcoves that would become my home for the next couple of hours.

The room was brightly lit and sterile. Each room had a boxy, stiff, and well-worn recliner for the patient to use and an uncomfortable cafeteria type chair for the caregiver. This was not designed to provide a Zen experience!

It was more like a production line.

The chemo nurses were all very cheerful and efficient. They asked me a series of questions about side effects, documented all my vital numbers, discussed the drugs I was taking, and praised me for doing well. Then they put what looked like a disposable diaper on the arm rest, pulled out several packages of one-time use supplies and started poking my veins on my arm or hand to prepare the IV. Once I was set, they left for the pharmacy to grab my special cocktails.

About five minutes later, they returned to yell, "Chemo check!"

Instantly, another nurse would come into the room and ask the same questions each time: *what is your name? when were you born?* Once the chemo was confirmed and the ok given, the nurse put on a full covering rubber gown and rubber gloves so that she could work with the chemo. Those kinds of precautions just drove home how dangerous chemo is.

We just had to repeat the process for the next bag. When I had three bags of chemo, it took about three hours, and with only two bags, it took about two hours. That was your inside look into the chemo treatment regimen.

I was embarrassed to see people who were aware of my cancer but I hadn't seen in a while because I didn't *look* the part. They were forever shocked to see me because nothing had changed about my outward appearance. They were expecting a frail person, riddled with disease, and beaten down by cancer, not an active and healthy-looking man. I have my hair, I'm tanned from hiking, golfing, and surfing, and I even gained two pounds.

Note: my weight fluctuated in a 10-pound range as I entered into and recovered from chemo treatments during any given month.

Though you wouldn't know it to see me, the treatments were still difficult. After two sessions with one fewer bag of chemo, I came to believe that the net change was negligible.

I continued to struggle with chemo brain, nausea, and fatigue after Healing Fridays. I found it interesting that the intensity of the ill feelings appeared to be less, while the duration was longer. I discovered that I did much better in the morning with the afternoons being relegated to naps and nausea. I became very active in the mornings, taking full advantage of my good moments.

I look at my cancer as a gift. I know that is crazy, but if I can help others take a conscious and realistic look at what is important in their lives and have them find more joy, create better relationships, and make a positive impact on their community, then my cancer *is* a gift. Sure, it stinks to have to deal with the "healing" every three weeks but I know I have two good weeks to look forward to. We are all going to say goodbye at some time so in that way, I was no different than anyone else. All I could do was live in the moment and ease the journey for others.

Many people were inspired by my mindset. For those who know me well, my outlook was not surprising. I had a conversation in Boulder four years ago. I was sharing my beliefs about life, about people, and about my impact on others. There were two gentlemen that I did not know and my very dear friend, Linda Hughes, sitting at the table. These two gentlemen were calling *BS* on my optimism and belief that good can come from almost any place.

"No, this is who Les is, you could both learn from him," Linda said.

I found myself wondering if I *was* full of BS. I did a lot of soul searching during that time and concluded that, no, that is just who I am and, frankly, I like that about myself.

Coming full circle, there I was living the life I believed in and hopefully, inspiring others on the way.

Despite my optimism, I was frustrated by the lack of consistency and improvement in my response to chemo. I was hoping to have at least some of the side effects diminish with the dropping of one bag of chemo. It didn't look as though that was going to happen. The side effects were changing, not improving. Allow me to explain.

The overall nausea, tiredness, and flu like symptoms diminished in intensity but increased in duration. Under three bags, I was feeling fine by the Wednesday after "Healing Friday." When we switched to two bags, the impact lasted almost a full two weeks! The most significant of the symptoms were "chemo brain" (a fogginess that doesn't seem capable of lifting), dizziness (I had to stand in the shower holding myself up with both hands), and fatigue (I often took two naps on Wednesday simply because I couldn't keep my eyes open). It was crazy but I had to conclude that the cancer was having no impact and 100% of the yuckiness came from the cure!

I felt much better from 5:00 a.m. until noon each day. After noon, the sickness descended. It was as if a switch had been flipped turning high energy and clear headedness into severe fatigue and confusion. I was blessed to have the ability to schedule my workouts and most of my appointments in the morning. Afternoons would have to be devoted to catching up, occasional appointments, naps, and relaxation.

One of my favorite activities was playing my ukulele in the afternoons. With the struggle of the chemo treatments, I just didn't have the gumption to play. I missed it, but I kept talking myself out of it. I needed to find a way to make my playing a social thing with friends so that I would attend to it more often.

DRUGS

One of the most interesting things about this journey is the massive amount of science, research, and treatments that are being developed and refined every day. One drug, Keytruda, is rather new on the market. There is plenty of good information out there about Keytruda. The drug has only been available for about seven years and the results are phenomenal. Stage IV lung cancer had a 5% five-year survival rate before Keytruda. Since its introduction, the five-year survival rate is trending towards 25%. I imagine that as time goes by those percentages will be even better and perhaps the ten-year survival rate will rise to 25%. I was not looking just to survive, however. I was looking for a ten-year "thrival" rate!

The mental side of cancer and our healing treatment were challenging. By the time two weeks passed and I finally started to feel better, my mind immediately began wondering about the following Friday. The closer I got, the more I started to dread it and began ruminating about the awful sensations that were sure to follow. For the most part, I could control my thoughts, but man, those little buggers kept finding a way into my consciousness.

So much for maintaining the "perfect" positive attitude.

BACK IN THE CHEMO CHAIR

I was sitting in the chemo chair, having just been hooked up to my first bag of juice. We were on about my 10th treatment. It was probably the easiest part of the process, as all I had to do was sit back and read my books. I was trying to create a consistent life plan for the three-week intervals of medication and recovery, but the chemo didn't seem to get the memo. Suddenly, the side effects lingered for the entire down time, giving me no break from one cycle to the next. It was mainly bouts of nausea, periods of fatigue, and constipation. Nothing I couldn't live with. I would just have to adjust my plans and my expectations.

I had two startlingly bad days, both taking place a week after the last chemo treatment and both the same. I woke up to severe sweating. When I tried to stand up, I found that I could not manage it without holding onto something. It was as if I was experiencing severe vertigo. In both situations, I struggled into the shower but could not wash myself because I had to hold the walls with both hands to remain upright. I sat for about a half hour until my equilibrium stabilized. I found myself so weak that it was a struggle to even open my eyes, and the weakness remained all day. I took two naps and went to bed early on both days. The strange thing was, I felt strong and normal on both the day before and the day after.

I added a new treatment to my regimen: lymphatic drainage massage. This is a massage process that focuses on the lymph nodes to help "unclog" them so that they can continue cleaning the impurities out of my body, improving my immune system, and helping the chemo work more effectively.

The therapist placed a white hand towel under my body so that she could capture the materials that drained from the lymph nodes. It was amazing how much "drainage" came out through my pores. I decided to keep it up for a few months to see if anything changed.

JUGGLING WORK AND CANCER

One of my Vistage groups gave me a director's chair as a gift at the retreat. Written on the back was: "Les Whitney, Master Chair." My life took two tracks, one for work and one for cancer treatments, appointments, and recovery activities. The next Healing Friday was a nonevent with a nap in the afternoon as the only side effect. Saturday and Sunday were both active days with few setbacks. Then along came Monday...

I woke up feeling great!

I felt good enough to attend my monthly meeting with my fellow Vistage chairs. We processed my issue, "What do I do with the rest of my life?" It was a high energy session that left me completely drained at the end. And this was when the true impact of the chemo treatment showed up.

I got home at 5:00 p.m. on Monday and went straight to bed. I woke up at 5:00 a.m. the next morning, went to the gym, and then back home for a nap at 7:30 a.m. I was up again at about 11:00 a.m. for lunch and then back to bed for my afternoon nap until 5:00 p.m. I stayed up until 9:00 p.m. and then went back to bed again. All told, I slept about 24 hours in a 32-hour period. I was rapidly coming to recognize fatigue as one of the leading side effects of the treatment. I also realized that there was no way of knowing how my body would respond from one chemo session to the next.

I ran my Key Executive group meeting on Wednesday and played golf on Thursday and then joined my CEO group for a retreat at the Ritz Carlton for the weekend. It was a great experience and very relaxing.

> *At times, I look at my cancer as a gift. I know that is crazy, but if I could help others take a conscious and realistic look at what is important in their lives and have them find more joy, create better relationships, and make a positive impact on their community, then my cancer is a gift.*

Our weekend speaker, Brett Pyle, asked each of us how long we thought we would live. This is a great exercise to give people perspective. Most people said thirty or forty years or more.

I told the group three years!

The faces of the group were frozen like characters in a wax museum. They expected me to be more optimistic and upbeat, until I explained my philosophy. You see, if I said ten or twenty years, then I would have plenty of time and I wouldn't need to make any decisions or any changes to my current lifestyle. However, if I said I was only going to live for *one* year, then my decision-making would become much more urgent. If I only had one year, I would quit everything, grab Teresa, and go see as much of the world as I could in the time I had left.

Three years was short enough to have a sense of urgency, but long enough that I wouldn't need to quit my work and flip my world upside down. Every morning, I could look at my life and my plans as having three years left from that day...a revolving three-year window. It was an easy philosophy for me to get my head around.

I put a great deal of thought into a presentation I was asked to develop. I planned to borrow the title of the Tim McGraw song, "Live like you were dying!" as the title of my presentation and perhaps this book. It fits with my three-year window and clarifies what my life might look like if lived as if I was dying. I was surprised that most of the decisions and actions I made daily were significantly impacted by living as if I were dying. Try it in your mind; you will be surprised at the results.

I went in for my fourth MRI of my brain and a PET scan of the rest of my body. I met with the doctors to hear how I was doing. The first meeting was with the neurological surgeon who did my brain surgery. He was almost giddy with excitement as he shared that there were absolutely no signs of cancer in my brain. He was also excited that I was responding so well to the chemo treatments. It seemed as if I had nearly all my function back in my left hand which meant there was a possibility I'd be able to regain the ukulele skills I so missed. That was great news!

I met with the pulmonary oncologist a few hours after. He was not inclined to get excited but did say that there was no sign of active cancer in my lymph nodes and only about 10% to 15% of my lung cancer was active, the remainder was scar tissue. You might think we would all be jumping for joy and high fiving each other, but that didn't happen. The doctor said this was very good progress, better than most, but that it didn't change anything in our program or in my prognoses.

He said, "you still have incurable lung cancer, and you will still need to continue the three-week chemo intervals for the rest of your life." He burst my bubble by telling us that I would be continuing the chemo and the immunotherapy forever, not just the immunotherapy. But seeing my dejection, he mentioned that we had the option to cut back the chemo to 75% of what it was then. This was only an option if I started having more severe side effects or if my blood numbers showed more damage to my kidneys and liver.

What all this meant to me was that we were making good progress and I was responding well to treatments (at least for now). What it also meant was that my life was as good as it was going to get for the foreseeable future...one tough post-chemo week and two relatively good weeks would be the best I could hope for.

Teresa was not one to tell me how challenging this journey had been for her. She simply took on each task, carrying things for me. She worried about our future without ever complaining or showing how the journey was impacting her. The only time I got a sense of what she was going through was when she talked with her friends. The woman is a stoic, but she's human.

I could not ask for a better partner in life.

Healing Friday was not as bad the next few times around, and I was hopeful things had changed. Then reality hit. We did my treatment and then went home to convalesce. Saturday morning, we drove down to Mexico to spend three days looking at the ocean while I recovered. I couldn't eat anything, my body ached all over, my head felt like it was full of cotton balls with pressure pushing from the inside out, and I had intense diarrhea (perhaps TMI?). We even tried to do our walk on Saturday, but two miles was all the energy I had. It was like my entire body was revolting against me.

Sunday and Monday remained the same. I was extremely fatigued. The effort to read was too much, so I just laid down and waited for everything to pass. Eating was a challenge as well; everything tasted like metal. Over the half year of initial treatments, I averaged a loss of about five pounds during the five recovery days. This time, I lost eight pounds in four days. I was just going to have to quit hoping for a better reaction on the next treatment. Note: I always gained the weight back during the next two weeks.

The balancing act between the volume of chemo and the side effects was constantly in motion. I had wrongly assumed that once we started, we would simply stick to the plan. However, with such wide swings of recovery, side effects, and inconsistent feeling, I quickly learned to be flexible.

On a positive note, I played the ukulele for about an hour and a half on Saturday and played the best I ever had since I lost the use of my left hand. I was so happy to have my ability to play back. Sadly, I didn't have the stamina to play again over the weekend.

On the work front, I was doing more and more of my meetings via FaceTime and Zoom. This was a godsend as it allowed me to remain effective and impactful without leaving the house. I could lie down between meetings, and I was more focused during the meetings. Teresa kept pushing me to do all my meetings that way.

TESTIMONIAL: JACK DALY

After being diagnosed and speaking out about cancer, I found more and more people with similar stories. One of them was Jack Daly, a Vistage speaker and author of ten bestselling books including *The Sales Playbook: For Hyper Sales Growth*. Both Jack and his wife walked down the same path as me. It ended tragically for her, and while Jack dealt with his grief, he was also dealing with his own illness. He said:

I met my wife as a sixteen-year-old in high school, and we had an unbelievable marriage of forty-seven years. In February of 2017, she was diagnosed with stage IV pancreatic cancer. We fought that battle but lost in November of 2017. I was a spectator on Les's journey, a very active and emotionally involved spectator, but a bystander, nonetheless. On April 1 of 2020, I was diagnosed with a malignant melanoma stage III on the top of my head. Within two weeks, they had me at the hospital, and took a slice off the top of my head about an eighth of an inch thick. They managed to get it all, and even fixed it so my hair would grow back.

I thought that was the end of it, but a year ago, it popped up again on my neck. I was on Keytruda for nine months and eventually, the prognosis was good. We can't find it anymore. It's interesting to have friends who are walking the same path. It helps to have people you can talk to. My journey has been calm compared to Les's, but I feel that kinship that only other cancer patients have.

THE NEW NORMAL | 127

LESSONS LEARNED: NEAR-TERM PLANS, ETERNAL GAINS

I'm going to hit it hard, because it's an important part of my mindset: I live like I've got three years left. No matter how healthy you are or what situation you find yourself in, you might want to reevaluate your own internal clock. How is your decision-making impacted if you see yourself living to 100? How many opportunities are you delaying if you don't perceive an expiration date on your life?

On the other hand, there's an old piece of advice that goes *seize the day, live like there's no tomorrow*. In that case, wouldn't we all call in sick to work, blow all our money on a party or a fancy vacation, and eat and drink to excess?

In between those two extremes is three years, where there is still time to plan, but not enough to get cold feet. Near term plans are things I can get behind and goals I can achieve without a lifetime to work towards them. Think vacations to exotic lands or traveling around your own backyard. It could be writing a novel or painting a landscape. It could be jumping out of an airplane if that's your thing or establishing a trust for your favorite charity. It's choosing what I want today rather than allowing others to make those choices for me or believing that I can always wait until tomorrow.

Near term plans do *not* include getting an advanced degree, starting a new company, or learning how to speak French. Those are very important things and a big part of my joy in life, pre-cancer. In fact, the future was my dream life, and I am a dreamer. It was painful to let go of some of those long-term goals, for sure. But I think I'm a better person for it.

By focusing on the immediate future, I am forced to make decisions about what is most important to me and my inner circle today. Teresa and I want to spend most of our remaining time together, meaning that we put more of an emphasis on things we can do as a couple. Travel, charity work, golf, and time with friends are all things we enjoy together. I may be interested in going to a NASCAR race (not really, but just an example), but if it's not something we can share, that doesn't meet the criteria.

One of the first things I suggest doing, after all the decisions about treatment and logistics are out of the way, is figure out what you want to do with the time you have left. The doctors may be saying six years, they may be saying six months, or even six weeks. No matter what the prognosis, don't let the treatments, the fear of dying, or the pain stop you from making short-term plans. It's your life and I encourage you to live every moment you've been given in the way that you want to the fullest level possible.

It has become a day-to-day journey with more good days than bad days.

What changes would you make in your life if you were on a similar journey? I looked and felt healthy. My mind was constantly reviewing all my options but making changes was difficult.

What would you be considering if you were in a similar situation?

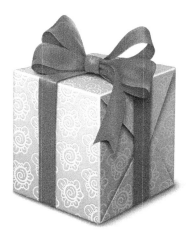

THE GIFT OF ACCEPTANCE

I've got stage IV lung cancer, and it is going to kill me! Accepting this fate has made my life so much richer.

I firmly believe that being able to accept a situation for what it is opens me up to many more possibilities than if I denied its existence. Too many people spend their energy wishing for a better past. This is wasted energy. We cannot change the past. We cannot change our situation as it exists. We can only live in the moment and change our behavior in anticipation of a better tomorrow.

I am going to have one bad week out of every three weeks. I can take action to try and ease the discomfort, but I cannot change what chemo does to me. That said, my two weeks of feeling great are filled with possibilities. I can focus on all that I can do. I don't mourn the things that cancer and age have taken away, rather I chose to find all the activities and opportunities that remain available to me.

Life is too short to allow limitations to stop me from living. I accept them. I chose to live with what is possible.

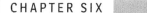 CHAPTER SIX

LIFE'S EBB AND FLOW WITH CANCER

Nearly a year into treatments, my activities, lifestyle, and chemo began to become more routine. It seemed as if the most consistent aspect of the three-week cycle was that some sort of symptom would show up each day. I didn't know what the symptom would be; I just knew it would be there.

The good news was the symptoms were more of a nuisance than problematic. For example, one new symptom has been leaky nose and leaky eyes. It appears there was always a drop hanging from the end of my nose or tears rolling down my cheeks. I went through a box of tissues a day. I also had to put Vaseline on my nose to relieve the chaffing and cracking. This became a problem during golf when tears would blur my eyes while I leaned over a putt, and then a drop would fall from the tip of my nose and make a direct hit on my golf ball...splat!

The most annoying impact was the significant reduction in my energy level. I had always been known for high energy (perhaps too much energy), but I was running out of gas every day. Historically, I would thrive on 6 1/2 to seven hours of sleep per night, but after chemo I absolutely needed ten hours. One week, I struggled to get my ten hours and found myself taking a nap during my Vistage group meeting while the guest speaker was presenting. It was probably not the most professional thing to do, but I had no choice. I decided that being present in whatever capacity I could was more important than keeping up a professional appearance.

The common symptoms—thinning hair, nausea, fatigue, no appetite, metallic taste, etc.— were nothing that couldn't be tolerated. A special thank you to Vistage speaker Jason Hartanov whose excellent presentation on overcoming limiting beliefs reminded me that I could do whatever I put my mind to, even with cancer. Occasionally, I found myself coming up with reasons why I couldn't live a full and fulfilling life. Jason's presentation brought me back to the right mindset where I could accomplish my dreams.

BACK FROM THE ABYSS

I didn't realize I was in the abyss until several days passed...

For whatever reason, I quit being me for two weeks. I lost all desire to do just about anything. I found myself not wanting to talk to anyone, not returning emails and phone calls, and not doing much of the planning and organizing work I needed to do in my job. I would sit down to read a book or article and could not get beyond two sentences. I would sit down to play the ukulele and quit after five minutes. I found myself going to bed between 6:00 p.m. and 8:00 p.m.

This was anything but intentional. I didn't realize I was putting everything on hold. My life became something I didn't recognize, and I didn't realize it in the moment.

When I look back, I guess I just got tired of having cancer and chose not to deal with it anymore.

Fortunately, I recognized how I was acting and accepted that I had changed.

Time to bounce back.

Then, surprisingly, the three days after my next chemo session were the best days I had since my diagnosis. I had more energy than I could remember having, my brain was clear (no chemo brain fog), and I did not have a moment of discomfort or nausea for a week. The bottom line was, I was feeling no ill effects from the chemo nor cancer.

Inside, I was celebrating! I was returning to being me. It was as if my body decided to remind my brain of who I was.

In response to my excitement, chemo decided to show me who was in charge. The next chemo session started about the same as all the others. Healing Friday was not a bad day, with just a little fatigue that afternoon. Saturday and Sunday were good exercise days (about seven miles per day walking) and I was able to rest comfortably both afternoons. We even tried to play nine holes of golf on Monday morning after chemo. After Monday morning, I became a zombie for the next two and a half days struggling to keep my eyes open, pushing myself to get up out of my seat, and ignoring everything else.

My blood was checked every Thursday before Healing Friday. There were about twenty to thirty numbers they checked every time. Some tests checked how the kidneys were handling the chemo, others checked the liver, red and white blood cells, hemoglobin, and more. The last time my liver numbers were inflated. It wasn't enough to worry the doctors, but enough for me to take action. The nurse said it was probably due to dehydration. When I told her I had enjoyed a beer after each round of golf, she was shocked!

"You are joking, right?" she cried. "You should not be drinking at all!"

Insert emoji with red cheeks.

Now, the literature I read said one or two drinks is not bad...I guess I was just using selective reading to determine my actions. So, the next time I would drink more water than usual (I usually drank over a gallon a day) and I would not drink alcohol at all. I would check the numbers to see if they improved. Once I got these new data points, I would make behavioral decisions going forward.

Teresa and I were finally taking a big trip, a bike and barge trip in Holland. We flew during what has traditionally been one of my toughest days. We decided to fly business class so I would have a pod with a bed. My thinking was that I would spend the day in bed anyway, so I might as well do it on the airplane. This would be a test to see how we do with international travel. If all went well, there would be more international trips in our future.

The next cycle rolled around before I knew it. There were blood tests on Thursday and then another Healing Friday. It was sad to think I would be leaving a state of health and vitality for a few days, yet I found joy knowing that I would be back to feeling great by the following Wednesday or Thursday!

That Wednesday, we flew to Amsterdam. It was a test of:

1. Identifying the soonest I could travel after "Healing Friday"
2. Experiencing, how well I could handle the joys of air travel: the jet lag and the crowds in Europe

3. Determining how my body would stand up to a week of cycling and sightseeing

If all went well, I assumed the next year would be a year of travel and adventure for Teresa and me.

THE CONVERSATION

I'd like to share some thoughts on "The Conversation." I've been blessed to speak with numerous people who have lost loved ones to cancer or some other awful disease. I've found it interesting that so many of those I've spoken with regret that they did not talk about all that they love and appreciate about each other nor what would be "next" after the disease took their loved one away.

The first and most prevalent reason people have explained for not having these conversations is they felt like talking about it would be a sign of giving up. The reality is, we are all going to die, so talking about what's next should be an annual conversation regardless of health status. I wanted to know that Teresa would be ok if and when the worst case happens.

I was also postponing talking to the people in my world about how grateful I was for their contributions to my life, letting them know the impact they have had on me, and simply letting them know that I love them. Again, the belief was that by approaching the subject of an "after I die," I would be giving up.

- Shouldn't I let people know how important they are to me all the time?
- Shouldn't I thank people for how they have influenced and molded me?

- Shouldn't I clean up all the unspoken conversations?
- How else could I ensure there would be no clouds hanging over my healing years?

Now is as good a time as any to engage with all the people who have made a difference in my life. In fact, if I can be completely honest with all my important conversations, the next ten healing years will be exponentially more joyful.

Finally, making sure that all the legal, estate, and trust work is complete is an important task to undertake. Too many of us believe we have plenty of time to take care of this business later. I have a much greater peace of mind knowing that Teresa and I have completely redone our estate plan and wills. Please, follow my lead, get your affairs in order, and have the conversations.

I'm reminded of an exercise I did years ago with my CEO groups. It was called the *Green Box Exercise* first shared by Adrian Geering of TEC Australia. It was time for Teresa and me to fill our Green Box, and perhaps others would like to create their own Green Box. Here is the exercise:

Jim McArthur was a TEC (a peer networking group that eventually became Vistage) Australia member. His father John was also a TEC member. John called his son Jim to let him know that he'd be flying to New Zealand the following day to try to close an important business deal. Jim, a pilot in the Air Guard Reserves, warned his father that potential typhoons could make travel hazardous. John laughed and reminded Jim that if anything tragic happened, to remember to get the "Green Box" out of the closet in his bedroom.

The next day, John was killed when his plane crashed into the side of a mountain on the north island in very low visibility. Several days after the funeral, he remembered his father's words about the Green Box. He called his mother, and they brought the Green Box to the family attorney. Inside, they found 28 envelopes. Here are the labels on the envelopes:

- Letter to my wife
- Letter to each child (3)
- Letter to the employees
- Letter to my mother / father
- List of most important 5 employees in the company & their strengths/weaknesses
- Off balance sheet deals
- Organizational chart
- Details of any company trusts
- List of personal and businesspeople that should be contacted in the event of passing
- Deals in process and evaluation of them
- Strategies that I was thinking about but hadn't told anybody
- List of trusted advisors and their roles (may or may not be currently working with company) such as attorney, accountant, etc.
- Instructions not addressed in will
- Copies of POA documents
- Copy of passport and birth certificate
- Copy of all credit cards
- Copy of physical property titles
- Personal stock portfolio information

- Details of life insurance—personal and company owned
- Details of all other insurance
- Copies of personal property valuations (jewelry, guns, collectables, etc.)
- Computer passwords
- Personal financial statement
- Extra passport photos
- Medical/Dental charts
- Funeral/Burial instructions
- Mementos and to whom you'd like them given

HOLLAND, AUGUST 2019

We flew to Holland the Wednesday after Healing Friday and the flight went surprisingly well. I wore a hospital mask on the flight to limit my exposure to the recirculating air. We wiped down our entire pod with sterile wipes, and slept the entire way to Amsterdam. It was a peaceful, uneventful flight and I felt great throughout.

The bike and barge trip was fantastic!

You've probably seen the iconic views of Holland in film, magazines, or maybe in person. The place is well suited for cycling as the entire country is crisscrossed with bike paths. Everyone in that country cycles so the paths in the city can be quite chaotic. But once we exited the city, the scenery and the travel were relaxing and beautiful. There was water everywhere, windmills turning, majestic green fields crisscrossed with dikes and canals, and swans greeting us at many turns. It was total peaceful splendor.

Unlike my body.

My body was not the same, of course. Before my cancer, I was exceptionally fit and full of energy. Now, as I crisscrossed the bridges and gently bicycled around Holland, I was no longer the physical specimen I had been before cancer. Short thirty-mile bike rides that I used to do effortlessly, now taxed my endurance. Teresa and I even skipped a day's ride to give me more time to recuperate. One afternoon was a little scary as I struggled with dizziness over the last five miles, and I had trouble keeping my eyes open. It wasn't even a strenuous ride, but my body just wasn't what it had been pre-chemo. I was learning to accept this as my new normal.

I didn't like it, but I accepted it.

I experienced some emotional turmoil on our bike and barge trip. The third morning was raining hard, so Teresa decided to stay on board while the rest of us rode our bikes. About noon that day, I pictured Teresa sitting alone, looking out at the world from the boat. For only the second or third time since I was diagnosed, something unusual happened.

I started crying.

I pictured Teresa traveling on her own after I was gone, and it just made me so sad. I knew she would be fine, she had lots of friends to support her and travel with her, it just wouldn't be me. I was not saddened by potentially dying from cancer, I was saddened by the thought of missing years with Teresa. But that kind of thinking didn't help, and I knew I should focus on all the benefits of my condition, and enjoy the beauty of life.

The trip did so much for my psyche. I learned that I could travel comfortably and, with the proper precautions, safely. If I flew business class, wore a face mask, and cleaned my seat area, I could be relatively sure I wasn't making things worse. I was also careful about eating foods that other people may have touched like sliced cheese at the cheese farm, anything in a buffet, or anything open to handling. It was easy once it became a habit.

We made the decision to move our chemo appointment from 9:30 a.m. to 12:30 p.m. It begged the question, what to do with this new found free time? Have fun? We started the morning with a one-hour gym session, then went out to breakfast before teeing off for golf at 7:00 a.m. We finished golf at 10:30 a.m., then went for coffee and pastries before going to chemo.

I continued to have these feelings of being a cancer fraud because the good times outweighed the bad times.

I read some updated statistics about my wonderful cancer. Unfortunately, the information was not good, but it did leave room for outliers like me. I was confident we would outperform all the other cancer patients. The scary thing was that my cancer still had only a 5% five-year survival rate. They were finding the short-term (1 year) survival rate remaining at 50% even with adding immunotherapy (Keytruda). I have to believe they did not have a sufficient sampling of the five-year rate to let us know if that had improved.

There is so much information about everything, nowadays. Be very mindful of what you search for, the sources, and details. Health science is still in its infancy. There is much we don't know, and every person's situation is unique.

Some of the articles I read were a little disheartening in that they indicated that no matter how well I reacted to the cancer treatments, the results could change overnight. Apparently, the combo of chemo and immunotherapy worked very well all the way up until it stopped working. Teresa and I remained positive. We knew that we could tolerate the five days of discomfort around the chemo. We knew that we could enjoy the days in-between. And we knew that I was unique and would outperform all the projections because, "that's just what we do!"

We were scheduled for another CT scan and then we would meet with the doctor a few weeks later. I held out hope that everything would be cleared up and we could just remain in maintenance mode. But I had waking nightmares that we were going to discover that my body was riddled again with cancer.

There was a reason for this, just a little pessimism leaking into my psyche. The plan with the doctor was to discuss cutting back on the chemo to make the five days afterwards easier. That was something I was not interested in if it was going to compromise the efficacy of my treatment. However, if the liver damage would be too much, then maybe we should cut back. We also wanted to discuss some new targeted testing Teresa read about that works with simple blood tests. I contacted the company that created this approach, and they informed me they no longer work directly with patients, and we must go through our insurance carrier. I planned to discuss this with the doctor and then either have Kaiser order the tests or I would go out and do it myself. The cost of the test was about $5,000; a small price if it could lead to better results.

Lung cancer is so different from the other cancers. I knew of several people who were diagnosed with cancer around the same time I was who were either in remission and not receiving treatment or no longer with us. It seemed there was an end date for most treatments but no end date for stage IV lung cancer treatment. It was depressing to limit my plan to living in the chemo cycle forever. I was making the most of it, even jetting off to Hawaii for some time to mentally escape.

On a humorous note, I mentioned before that I didn't ever throw up (gross). We discovered that when the nausea became so intense that I thought I might throw up, I sneezed instead. Hard! Once that happened, all the bad nausea feelings disappeared. Weird!

HAWAII

After Wednesday of healing week, I could completely forget that I had cancer. In this lull, I had no symptoms and no indications that anything was going on with me physically or mentally. This allowed Teresa and I to enjoy every day in Hawaii without limitations: working, golfing, exercising, eating, and simply having fun.

Life couldn't get any better. (Except for the cancer thing)

We enjoyed Maui; it was beautiful. We played golf on the first day with one of my Vistage members who was finishing his family vacation. Two days later, we had dinner with friends from the gym and garden club who were there for a three-day birthday trip. We could travel around the world and still run into friends! How great was it that our cancer-impacted lifestyle was becoming normal?

When we returned from Hawaii, we met with the doctor to discuss my latest CT scan and the results had me a bit baffled. My oncologist was pleased, almost excited, to tell us that nothing had changed! The lung tumor was the same size as it was after the last scan. I found this sobering. How could he be excited about no improvement? Once again, I realized that he had no expectation of "curing" my cancer with the treatments that were available but was excited that it had not gotten worse.

"Everything is working!" my doctor proclaimed. "I couldn't be more pleased with the results. Compared to other patients, you are doing amazing!"

What was he excited about?

Two things: first, the cancer was controlled for the time being and second, I was handling the side effects of chemo better than most. My five days of misery after infusion were easier than what others experienced. My white and red blood cell counts had not fallen out of the normal range, and even the fact that my liver numbers were inflated was not a concern as typical cancer patients struggle to maintain good blood numbers.

As a competitive person, I found it hard to celebrate status quo. The idea that we were simply trying to extend my life and give me a good lifestyle in the process really hit home. If I could keep managing the side effects and as long as the cancer remained static, my new way of living would remain unchanged. The prayers I needed at that time were for a new miracle cure to come along before my maintenance program ran its course. Every day we heard about new progress in cancer treatments. From "liquid biopsy" that would allow for finding targeted therapy through blood samples to a new cure for pancreatic cancer that mutates cancer cells into killing themselves, these were some of the amazing advancements. We could only hope that the researchers would find the same type of cure for lung cancer.

Teresa was constantly researching and she found a surprising "cure." It is something you could buy off the shelf at your local specialty store. In fact, this cure has become so popular that most stores quickly went out of stock and prices have risen three to five times in three months. What is this miracle and where can you find it?

Dog dewormer. Found at your local pet store.

We had a friend who was very ill, and the prognosis was not good. She started on dewormer and saw significant progress in her breathing and her tumors shrunk (at least that was the story she shared). I was not quite ready to go down this path... but who could tell what tomorrow would bring. I surmised taking dog dewormer wouldn't have any downside. (Unless I developed a strange desire for milk bones and sniffing everyone who walked past me)

DISCLAIMER: My guess is that most of this is made up. Please do not go out and buy anything just because you read it here (or online for that matter). Talk to your doctor and if they give you the okay, try it out. I am just including it because it makes a good story.

The impact of my altered state really hammered home one Friday. During my chemo induced haze, I booked flights to Colorado and Washington. The trips were from different airports. I told Teresa that we were flying out of John Wayne during our trip to Colorado. When we arrived to check in, we were informed that our flight was from LAX. In my altered state, I mixed up the two trips causing us to cancel and miss our dear friend's wedding. This was one of many commitments I missed since starting chemo. I always used my near photographic memory as a tool in my leadership. Sadly, this skill was gone forever.

Closing in on 20 chemo sessions, I was starting to dread Healing Friday. Knowing that I was going to lose one out of every three weeks was depressing. I was trying to push through and hoped that it was just a phase. I needed to redefine what healing week meant to me so that I could accept the pain and discomfort.

Throughout this journey, I kept finding people in my life who were struggling with cancer. It seemed like there wasn't a person in America who was not touched. My friend informed me that her sister had lung cancer and that it was compounded by a serious cough, up to and including coughing up blood. She did not handle her first chemo session well. Her sister told me she was talking seriously about quitting chemo and allowing the cancer to take its course. I have not spoken with her since so I don't know if she gave up. I do know that there have been a few days when giving up has crossed my mind.

DECEMBER 2019

A year had passed since discovering my brain tumor. Remembering what life was like pre-cancer was beginning to be a challenge. I hoped we could continue to have good results. It was quite the year for Teresa and me, one that we would not wish on anyone, but a year that brought us closer to each other than we ever could have dreamed.

We had Healing Friday just before Christmas, then ran off to convalesce at a friend's home in Palm Desert. Since the previous two chemo sessions were miserable, I thought I would try a new approach. I had been given Zofran for nausea, but I didn't take it very often since I really didn't get nauseated that severely or for any measurable length of time. I realized, however, that when I took Zofran, the chemo brain, aching body, fatigue, and overall malaise were significantly diminished. I asked myself, *why wait for nausea to use Zofran, just take one in the morning, and see what happens?*

I did that on Tuesday and Wednesday and had the best post chemo Tuesday and Wednesday yet. I worked out, played golf, went to the movies, and felt great all day both days. It was *amazing!* Next chemo session, I was determined to take a pill every day to see what would happen.

I had about twenty chemo sessions so far, more than a year of treatments! I heard so many stories of people who ended chemo after three, five, or ten sessions and then they were determined to be in remission. I envied them a little as I looked ahead to five or ten more years of chemo. Perhaps it was appropriate that I would be the person who had to show up every three weeks for chemo, since my vision for myself before cancer was to become the "sage" or "village elder" who people seek out for wisdom and guidance. I imagined myself becoming the "chemo elder," guiding new and struggling patients through their cancer journeys and perhaps even finding a way to lighten their burdens as they fought this evil foe.

TESTIMONIAL: VICTORIA KORTLANG

Victoria is my sister. The longer we have known each other, the closer we have become. My cancer really resonated with her not only as a family member but also as a person struggling with her own health issues. Vicky said:

I was two and a half when Les was born. We didn't see eye to eye very often, especially as teenagers. We used to fight all the time. It took me a long time to realize that I was jealous of Les. He was good looking, he always had a tan, and he was into sports. And I was a chubby older sister, who just watched TV and stuff. He was the apple of our parents' eyes. I never thought we'd become close, but now we are.

The biggest impact he had on my life was by helping me express myself. I was very shy and introverted. He just pushed me, he always said the right things: "Sis, I'm so proud of you" and things like that.

One of my fondest memories was when Les, Teresa, Johnny (my husband), and I went on a Mediterranean cruise. Les has always been a world traveler. We had traveled to Mexico and Central America in the past, but this was our first trip into Europe. Les was so sure of himself. He got to the hotel the night before we did. And he and Teresa met us on the pier, getting off the water taxi.

He said, "Okay, we're going to go put away your suitcases. And then you're not going to sleep. You're not going to sleep. You have to see Venice!" He took us all over Venice walking everywhere. We spent the entire day, and it was just fabulous. He was our tour guide, and he knew it all. We had a wonderful day that day and wonderful cruise.

When he found out he had cancer, Johnny and I wanted to spend a day with him. We also wanted to be there to support Teresa while Les was getting his brain surgery. So, Les and Teresa invited us to spend the day with them. We went to breakfast, and we got our nails done. He decided we needed to get our nails done. It was fun and we just had a lovely day. You would never have thought that he was going to go through what he went through, and even that was easy. Les just made all of it easy. I know he has lousy days after his chemo. And I know there's been other things that have been rotten, but that man is so positive. I don't want to lose my brother. I don't want Teresa to lose her husband. But Les helps all of us get through it. I'm just so proud of him.

When he found out he had cancer, I went on a major self-improvement campaign. I joined the food addicts' group and lost a lot of weight. My husband and I sold our house that we had lived in for 46 years. We never would have left there, or found the courage make the move without him. I would say to anyone reading this: if you want to do something, do it. Live your life. Live it fully.

LESSONS LEARNED: FOCUS ON WHAT TRULY MATTERS

One of my strengths, and what I hope to share with you, is how I can very quickly go from experiencing something stressful to thinking about how I can make it joyful. It's a mindset. How can I make this great? There's no one answer. But several things are important. Living every day to the fullest, fitting in your interests, and putting the focus on people you care about will change your experience from negative to positive.

I love to travel. That matters to me, so I think of ways I can fit that into my life. I have a number of people that I love, so I'm trying to make sure to prioritize time spent with those folks. And I want to give back. I want to help others achieve the greatness within them. That's what brings me joy. And so, the question becomes, how can I do more of that? In the short amount of time I have left, how can I really focus on what matters?

When I was first diagnosed, and I started my blog, right away I got feedback from people saying that they appreciated the honesty in my writing. By the end of the first month, I knew I had to find a way to help cancer victims. Most people don't handle this the way I do, but it's a much better place than where a lot of people find themselves. By focusing on what matters and eliminating excess tasks, you can take your stress level down a notch. Even with the disease, if you can give up a job that's bringing you down or get out of a toxic relationship, it will clear the way to a better life. I don't have much time left. I can't get bogged down in things that don't bring me joy.

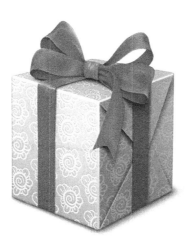

THE GIFT OF CLARITY

How can you, regardless of your situation, gain more clarity in what is meaningful and important in your life?

While blogging certainly helped, writing this book was even more impactful. Under the guidance of my publisher, he encouraged me to not only document my journey and bring in some behind the scenes ideas, but to ask others for their perspective.

Clarity is a funny thing. If I focus only on myself, I will achieve one level of clarity, that may be considered wise given my circumstances. True clarity, however, need not be singular nor absolute. The responses to my blog have brought an even deeper level of clarity around what is important.

When I focus on the moment, the moment is there and it's all I will ever have. The past is a distant memory, bouncing around in my brain. The future is equally intangible... merely my imagination at work. The ability to focus on the present is powerful.

But so is focusing on the why.

- Why document this?
- Why keep working?
- Why invest time in others?

In my case, I love people so much, I can't imagine not having them around (within boundaries). But part of this is also living my own truth. I can't share wisdom I don't have. So, instead of making it about me for a moment, I think if anyone can find those things that fill them up with joy, then all other areas of their lives will be meaningful. Rather than worry about dying, I look at how can I feel as good as possible on the days between chemo. How can I fill those days with joyful things? How can I have a positive impact within my community? How can I invest more in the things that I really value?

To me, that is living. And that is clarity!

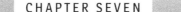 CHAPTER SEVEN

A NEW NORMAL

Throughout the second year of my treatment, time and events started to become as one. After about 25 treatments, both my oncologist and my brain surgeon raved about how well the initial surgery worked, how well the chemo was working, and about how well I was handling the entire process. They both made a comment that, when I was diagnosed with stage IV lung cancer, their expectations of me being alive today were not very high. They both reminded me that, even with current technology, the survival rates were not good.

The oncologist said that the clock for how long I would survive was turned off! He said that there was "no expiration date" on me going forward. As long as I continued to handle the process well, we could have every expectation that I would be writing these posts five years later.

It was almost a miracle.

And yet, with all these happy thoughts, I still wanted to be the captain of my life. I wanted to know what was going to happen every moment so that I could remain in control. I wanted to be able to plan when I would need to stop and when I could be active. But it didn't work that way.

Using the Zofran more freely during the last cycle made a significant difference in how I handle the really bad times. What it didn't do was help me control when the bad times showed up.

It had become abundantly clear that my worst day was Monday after Healing Friday. Monday became a day of nothing. It drove me crazy as I wanted to plan the good times, mediocre times, and bad times. I wanted to be the boss of my cancer and my cancer was not cooperating. Because I no longer had an expiration date (a budding mindset), I had plenty of time to figure it out. I just needed to determine what I was figuring out.

Giving up was not an option.

Cancer could not define me, but it did inform how I needed to spend my life. We were doing a great job of working with the three-week cycle and managing health, work, fun, and learning. We had to keep working to let me maintain control. I was excited to dream that I would be working with the amazing men and women in my Vistage group for as long as they would have me. I found a rhythm to work and life that made everything doable. Teresa and I would continue to thrive and continue to improve our relationship throughout the process. The hope of additional years would allow me to help many more people and use my cancer to have a greater impact on the world.

I'm constantly reminded that I have to continue the chemo and immunotherapy treatments for the rest of my life (or until they find a less invasive way to control the cancer or, better yet, they find a cure). To ease my anxiety, my oncologist said that we could be flexible with my treatments. For example, we could just do immunotherapy occasionally, (i.e., before a major trip) and we could move the dates around and maybe do one session after four weeks and then next time after two weeks.

LIVING LIFE IN 2020

I was sitting in San Diego with eight hundred fellow Vistage Chairs and staff overflowing with well wishes and support from people who truly care about me. I felt compelled to share my gratitude. You may recall that I was in San Diego, with my fellow Vistage Chairs the previous year, when the neurologist called me to let me know that my brain tumor was more than just a single tumor and that, yes, I had stage IV lung cancer. This conference reminded me that my life was moving on within my new reality and yet so much of it remained unchanged.

Cancer could not define me, but it did inform how I needed to spend my life.

I arrived at the annual chair conference in 2020 feeling extremely grateful that my body had responded so well to all the treatments and that so many people had been a part of Team Whitney. The minute I walked into the conference, I was greeted with hugs, words of encouragement, and words of appreciation for sharing my journey. I don't think I have ever been hugged so much as I was hugged over those 48 hours. It seemed like every hug added days, weeks, or even years to my life.

I was fortunate to visit Maui in the spring with our niece Athena and her husband Manny to attend the wedding of our nephew Andy and his lovely wife Shirley. I was extremely blessed that they allowed me to officiate their wedding on the beach. Furthermore, their good friends Scott and Julie wanted to get married in Hawaii as well and allowed me to "marry" them while I was at it. How awesome that they would include me in the next chapter of their lives and that we would all be distracted from the ugliness of cancer, at least for a moment!

The trip did have an impact on my cancer journey, unfortunately.

The service was a Thursday afternoon before Healing Friday. It was followed by a luau as the reception. We joined in the luau but left about a half hour early to catch the redeye for California. We needed to arrive in Southern California early so that I could complete my pre-chemo blood test in the morning and my infusion in the early afternoon. Boy, was I whipped! To top it off, flying causes dehydration which meant I went into chemo dehydrated.

"Drink plenty of water" the doctors and nurses told me to mitigate the impact of the chemo. Starting off dehydrated seemed to make it tough to drink enough to catch up. Why am I sharing all of this? Because Monday, Tuesday, and Wednesday I just could not shake the fatigue and "chemo brain" symptoms. Foggy headed and desperately needing sleep left me frustrated, miserable, and angry. I felt like I couldn't get a break. These emotional swings were so unlike me and starting to drive me crazy. I expected to control my emotions and remain positive throughout.

I was no longer an athlete. This sounds strange for a 65-year-old to suddenly realize that he was no longer an athlete, but there I was. My abilities had diminished over the years; however, the last year hammered it home. I had lost my balance, my agility, my strength, and my endurance. The diminished capacity showed up in my poor golf game, my recent fear of surfing alone, and my inability to walk/ hike long distances. It was humbling and disappointing to have to change my view of who I was even if it was inevitable with or without cancer. It was as if all the aspects of aging were compressed by my program to control the cancer.

MY BRAIN

Because the brain seems to do its thing most of the time, I had taken it for granted. I always believed that my ability to think clearly was one of my greatest assets. Therefore, discovering that my brain did not want to function at all during chemo was frustrating and scary. Under chemo I could not even force myself to think on any topic. It was as if my brain was in a jar of formaldehyde suspended in space. It hurt to try and think. I reached in for a thought and returned with a handful of incoherent mush. It was scary to not be able to process anything. I just wanted to curl up in a cave completely removed from all humanity until I could function mentally.

It is almost like a rebirth the first morning I wake up after each chemo session with a clear head. I silently celebrated the reemergence of ME! every time I returned from the abyss of chemo brain.

Let's all celebrate ourselves. Our unique selves. Let's cherish the times when we can be so fully who we are, because there will be times when each of us loses that for a moment, a day, a week, or longer. Each of us has been given gifts that some of us take for granted. Get to know your gifts, regale in them, share them, and thank them for being part of you.

COVID-19, MARCH 2020, THE WORLD CHANGED!

My health issues paled compared to what was happening throughout the world. There was a pandemic sweeping the globe and, in every nation, people were under lockdown. I had not ventured outside of the home except to take walks since my chemo treatment on March 13. Like most Americans, I was going a little stir crazy. There was only so much reading, playing music, or watching TV that I could handle in a day. The lack of entertainment was compounded by the lack of sports to watch on TV.

From that day on, all meetings with clients, both individual and group, moved onto the internet. I was amazed at how easy and effective technology was for meetings. I suspected all of us would stay home a little more and work virtually even after this crisis had passed. I was also hearing about groups getting together virtually for happy hour. What a great way to stay connected! Perhaps we would even pull out our musical instruments and have a ZOOM JAM in the near future?!?

It was clear that in times like this, my little cancer issue was insignificant in the grand scheme of things.

A pattern was emerging. It seemed my reaction to each chemo treatment was a little worse than the time before, which was a little worse than the time before that, which was a little worse than... etc., etc., etc. These were not big changes. It was nothing I couldn't handle; I just wished it would get easier with experience rather than tougher. It was crazy this time because after filling my brain with volumes of cancer education, I was unable to absorb all the COVID-19 information. I felt like the world was changing and leaving me behind. Fortunately, once I came out of the chemo haze, I was able to catch up and became a coronavirus news junkie like the rest of America.

Kaiser postponed all MRIs and PET scans for the near future so I would not receive further updates on my progress for a while. With COVID-19 in our world (especially my immune-compromised world), I found that I was a little leery of other people. When walking, I found myself creating at least five feet of space between me and others when passing. There was a sense of foreboding when in the proximity of others. Teresa was not immune either. She still went out shopping (you could never have enough TP it seemed) and she delivered meals most days to the needy. When she returned, I avoided her until she showered and changed. Paranoid? Yes. It was better to be safe than sorry. I couldn't leave the house to get my hair cut, and I soon looked like I did in high school except the hair was white, not brown.

It was clear that in times like this, my little cancer issue was insignificant in the grand scheme of things. We were doing well, all things considered. How blessed we were to live in a time when someone like me could do my work via video conferencing. It seemed like the only thing that had changed work wise is that I didn't spend thirty to forty hours a month on the freeway. What a great benefit!

CEOs and business leaders were working hard to navigate this crisis, to care for their employees and their loved ones, and to find ways to thrive. My clients were finding ways to help each other navigate business challenges in a COVID-19 environment while most leaders tried to navigate the pandemic on their own. Many were finding ways to help in their communities, to provide opportunities for their employees, and to ensure that they would be able to recover quickly when the mess was over.

Business leaders get a bad rap from the media. I wished everyone could see these caring, loving human beings spending time and money to ensure the health, safety, and family security of their employees. One of my clients created a second shift to make face shields to *give* to medical workers and first responders. Another created a production line to make hand sanitizers. Another lost 100% of his revenue from March to the end of the year, yet he chose to pay all health insurance costs for those employees he had to furlough. Every Monday, I held Zoom meetings with my members so that they could help each other survive, thrive, and make an impact on their communities. It was truly magical.

Finally, I was able to schedule both CT scans and MRIs during the second half of the year. The results were the same, no change to the tumors. Once again, this excited the doctors, though for me it remained a downer to think that the only excitement coming from my cancer treatments was that it was still there and remained unchanged. It had not grown, nor had it shown up anywhere else. I asked the doctor if there was any chance that I would ever get off the chemo routine. He said only if my body could not handle the chemo. If that were to happen, we could get off for a session but no more. If I was to skip more than a few treatments, we would risk the cancer resurging. I brought this up to him because it seemed to take a little longer each time for me to recover from the chemo. Wednesday after chemo had now become the last day of discomfort.

I know I've mentioned it before, but it bears repeating. Whether you have cancer or know someone who does, every little gesture matters. Every thought, word, and deed makes a difference. Even listening in silence counts. I am so fortunate that after nearly two years of treatments, my community still engages with me on a daily basis. Add to their support Teresa's strength and perseverance. She shows up as more than my wife and caregiver, she's my best friend and my rock.

And that is not because she focused only on yours truly! Every day she went out to deliver food to older people (you know, our age) who were shut in. Yesterday, she went out to pick up a prescription for a woman. Thousands of Americans were stepping up and it made me proud to be an American and Teresa's husband.

At least we were exercising. We walked every day during the pandemic from four to six miles. I set up a gym in the back yard, so we could add variety to our fitness regime. To fill her time, Teresa went through all her old photo albums and scanned her favorite pictures. I had fun with the photos she shared with me as we relived memories from years and travels past. Traveling back through time never made me sad. It only strengthened our gratitude for our lives.

By May of 2020, I was doing fantastic. I was still quite cautious with social distancing, so much so that I was going stir crazy and decided to branch out a little. On Monday, we had dinner with our dear friends. It was our first outing since February, and it was so much fun, it took three days for the smile to finally fade from my face. We decided to head down to our Mexico house to convalesce from chemo, marking the first time we had been there since February as well.

Perhaps like you, our world was so different during COVID. Teresa was no longer allowed into the infusion room with me; everyone was wearing masks, and the medical staff had all the PPE on. It was kind of spooky! At least the commute to and from chemo was not bad with so few cars on the road. After over thirty chemo sessions, I got to the point where all the staff at Kaiser had become my friends which made tolerating the new COVID protocols easier. I was so grateful for their cheerful greetings and the joyful way they cared about all of us fighting cancer. I felt blessed that they were on my team.

Cancer and COVID were impacting my golden years in a negative way, however.

One week of sickness out of every three weeks, stuck inside the house every day with no gym, no travel, no dinners with friends, no sports to pass the time, life was reduced to the basics. It was just Teresa and me getting to know each other better and better. Who'd have thought we could learn more about each other in the past few months than after being together for nearly 40 years. Living with cancer made finding joy every day challenging...possible but challenging. For human interaction, I had Zoom. For exercise, I had the daily walk. For travel, I watched Rick Steves reruns. And to relax, I had books and the ukulele. It was not the life I planned but it was working for the time being.

I thought about death on and off. My thoughts drifted more to when it would happen, how I would feel as I become sicker, and how well I would be able to communicate with family, friends, and all the people who supported me.

- How could I say goodbye?
- How could I thank people for all that they have meant to me?
- How could I make amends to those I may have hurt?

I lived a good life with few regrets. I took pride in my accomplishments. In sports vernacular, I left it all on the court. I was proud of my relationship with Teresa. I was proud of the woman Athena (our niece who I view as a daughter) has become and hoped that I had a small part in her success. I was overwhelmed by the friendships and relationships that were so essential to my health and happiness.

In so many ways, I was blessed.

JUST SPOKE WITH THE DOCTOR, MAY 2020

We had our four-month meeting with the doctor, and he remained ebullient about the test results. There was no sign of new cancer activity anywhere in my body. The brain tumor was gone, and the lung tumor continued its slow demise. He also said that my risk from the COVID virus was no greater than his. He wasn't referring simply to the risk of contracting COVID, but the risk of bad results if I did get it.

In other words, I was about as healthy as a cancer patient could be.

So, what happened after experiencing his positivity? I had a particularly bad reaction to chemo after my next session. The fatigue, chemo brain, gurgling/angry stomach, and total body ache lasted all the way to Friday. Add to that, I had two short bouts of vertigo. For the first time since discovering my cancer, I fell into a deep depression. I was disappointed and disillusioned. I found myself focusing on all the things I was missing and losing in my life. My balance and coordination became worse and worse, I continued to fatigue easily, my eyesight diminished, my sleep was disrupted, I was stuck at home, and I felt as if I was not providing my clients/friends with the level of challenge and insight they had come to expect. All this pain was compounded by the agony of isolation because of COVID.

I began to consider making major changes in my life. Perhaps it was time to retire? I shared my thinking with two people: my special friend and concierge at Vistage (Kelly) and my close friend and past client Craig. Kelly told me that she began crying when she read my note and there would be a huge void in Vistage if I wasn't there. She said that if I could only give half of me, it was valuable and that I would be terribly missed. I can't remember Craig's exact words, but the gist of it was that my ability to impact people's lives and the difference I made had been invaluable to him and everyone he knew. I sat with both their comments for a day and came to a profound conclusion.

I realized I had lost clarity and focus. You see, my focus was way off. I had been thinking about everything I was

A NEW NORMAL | 163

losing rather than being grateful for all that I had. By now you realize that these feelings are so unlike me.

Clarity and a simple mindset shift brought joy back into my life. The time I spent with clients and friends was valuable. There were many physical things I could still do, perhaps not well, but I could still do them. I could still love and be loved. I could enjoy the two weeks I felt healthy each cycle and tolerate the one week of discomfort. It was not time to hang up all that I enjoyed; I just needed to understand that what I do and how I show up would be different.

A simple example of the mindset change was the round of golf I played the day after my epiphany. I often found myself getting angry and frustrated when I made a bad shot. But that day, every time I made a bad shot, I thought to myself, "Well, that was expected!" The joy in that mindset lead to Teresa and me having the most fun on the course since we learned of my cancer.

So many people rave about my positive attitude which I was proud to say had returned. Sadly, I also knew of cancer patients who didn't want to read my blog because they felt I was too positive. I believe it is important to share that I am human. I feel despair at times, I've just found a way to work myself out of it.

The bottom line was that retirement was off the table for now.

HEALING FRIDAY REACTION VARIABILITY

I had two chemo sessions in one month, and they could not have been more different. The first one was miserable, taking me a full seven days to recover from the infusion. It was challenging and depressing to wake up every morning feeling weak, achy, and cloudy headed. The second session was completely different. My worst day, as always, was Monday after chemo and I felt tired and a little achy. The next day, I felt about 90% normal and even well enough to enjoy dinner with our close friends (socially distanced of course). By Tuesday, I felt 100% and enjoyed a round of golf. I wish I could understand why this happens and, perhaps, find a way to control it.

My latest scans showed my tumor shrinking from 4.2 cm X 2.2 cm to 3.7 cm X 1.7cm. That was good progress. Again, I had to remind everyone (including myself) that the current strategy was not designed to cure me of cancer, simply to keep the cancer from doing any more damage. I could live twenty more years with cancer if it didn't grow or develop in other parts of my body.

> *Why use the word despair?*
> *I don't know any other word that describes my emotional state in the week following Healing Friday.*

I was closing in on my thirty-fifth treatment when I believed I would be dropping the chemo portion of my infusion cocktail and moving to immunotherapy only. My oncologist said that 90% of the miserable side effects were from the Alimta, not the Keytruda. Unfortunately, he saw no reason to make this change as in his mind I was handling the treatments extremely well. I would soon learn that the next change would not be what I expected.

We were hyper conscious of social distancing and staying safe during the pandemic. We still got out, just made sure we were being safe. I had no qualms about asking people to give me extra space, and I kept an even larger distance from those who didn't wear masks or those who wore masks halfway. My assumption was that anyone wearing masks incorrectly or not wearing them at all was much more likely to be infected with the virus.

TESTIMONIAL: LISA PAPINI

I knew Lisa through Vistage. She was hesitant to join at first because of her perception that it was an all-male club (It is not). I was able to help her at a difficult time in her life and then she was able to turn around and help me. Lisa says:

I am not a super religious person. I am not a person who even feels comfortable saying that out loud. But I believe with every shred of my being that God led me to Les.

In 2011, I was married with three children. Through a series of medical tests, my husband was diagnosed with stage IV prostate cancer. The only thing that they could do was prolong his life, not cure him. We had a six-year-old, a ten-year-old, and a twelve-year-old. I was working, and he was a stay-at-home dad.

For the next four years, he would have monthly checkups to see if the cancer had spread. And so we'd be up at Cedars Sinai Medical Center every single month. He passed away in November of 2015. I came out of that experience as a completely shell-shocked person who had huge anxiety problems and depression, but I still needed to show up every day for my kids and my job.

In about June of 2016, my cousin Matt suggested that I join Vistage. I had absolutely no interest whatsoever. Then I saw some people that were in a Vistage group that got to fly onto an aircraft carrier and all this great stuff. And I said, "All right, well, I'll talk to them." So, I came out and spoke with them. I was like, here's my deal. And I just kind of laid it all out there: I'm a widow. I'm here doing this. I'm trying to do that. Blah, blah, blah.

My cousin reached out to Vistage. And he said, "what do you have in our area?" And they referred us to Les. When I first met him, my shields were up. But I had a habit of going from shields up to brutally honest very quickly. I could do that instantly. I needed someone who could handle my shields and my honesty.

So, Les walked in the door, and we started talking. And I instantly said, "I'm a widow; my husband recently died. I'm kind of scared shitless. I'm trying really, hard. I think I'm doing a good job but I'm not sure."

He immediately said, "I hear you; you are not the only person that feels this way, the group can help you, you'll fit in, it'll be fine. People always do better as CEOs when they have a coach and peer group."

So, I said, "Alright, I'll give this a shot."

I joined in time for the Christmas meeting. I felt different from the others, but it all worked out fine. Over the next three to four years, I got to know Les. He is an extremely authentic person. He guided me out of the anxiety and depression that I was in. I was going to a therapist too, to deal with the loss of my husband. But Les taught me how to be a good CEO and good with my children. I basically have quite a few full-time jobs. The reason why I think it was God who brought us together is because at the time that my husband was diagnosed, all the way through the time that he passed, there were little things that happened in my life, things that Les would need to know.

For example, I have a best friend who is financially secure and has a great life. She has been my best friend since fourth grade. We haven't really been able to connect over like two years. And finally in 2011, we had a phone call. We talked for an hour, no problems. And then we said, "You know what, let's make this a regular thing." The next week my husband was diagnosed. So, by the time we had our next phone call, I was able to have that support. Little things like that happened so often that I recognized a pattern. I am so happy that can support Les.

I assumed that Les was a gift and that I was going to be forever in his debt and unable to pay it back. Then he got diagnosed with a very similar thing to what my husband had with no option for a cure. And instantly I thought, oh my God, this relationship is a two-way street. And it was my turn to guide him. The relationship turned into a fantastic partnership where at first I had been the recipient of all his support, and now we are supporting each other.

LESSONS LEARNED: PRIORITIZE AND ENJOY THE OPPORTUNITIES

We all see the world and interpret what happens in the world through our own lens. That lens is colored by our life experience, what we have learned from others, and our past interpretations of events. This became crystal clear when my oncology nurse said that he was glad that I would come into the chemo room cheerful and upbeat.

He said, "I know it is an act, but I appreciate it."

I thought to myself, *An act? This is who I am!* But as I strolled around the chemo ward dragging my IV hanger, I noticed that almost every other person in the room was sad, hurting, uncomfortable, and in a general state of malaise. I realized that this was his reality, and I didn't fit that reality, therefore I must be acting. This one observation had me striving to:

1. Suspend judgment and
2. Try to understand others' reality or truth.

Was I successful? Not as often as I would have liked. But I do know that when others judge or make comments, it says more about them than those they judge or comment on. I'm a dreamer. My entire life has been spent dreaming about and planning for whatever comes next. Cancer and now COVID have made dreaming difficult and disappointing. We cancelled several trips , first because of cancer and then because of COVID. It was hard to plan other trips when I didn't know when the world would open up. Actually, I found planning anything more than six months out impossible since I always wondered if I would still be alive. With my "three years to live" philosophy, it was hard to plan for a long-term future with Teresa. Should I make short-term decisions to maximize the time we had, or should I plan for the long haul and risk missing time, experiences, and enjoying the moment? It became a consistent experience weighing the short term over the long term and it colored every decision I/we made.

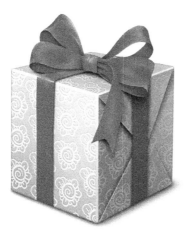

THE GIFT OF CHOICE

If you were sure you were going to die in one year, how would that change your decisions today? Would you put off that important conversation, time with loved ones, that trip of a lifetime, or that "I would love to do xxx sometime." I was always asking myself, "If not now, when?" What would I have to give up, what would I have to risk to make things happen sooner or even today?

As you can tell, living with cancer made me a bit more philosophical. I saw it as another benefit of having a terminal illness. Thinking about my life and striving for the best rather than just taking all the good and bad for granted allowed me to prioritize and enjoy the opportunities I did have. Awareness, appreciation, being present, excitement about little things, intense love, and more are all benefits of a cancer diagnosis.

When you embrace the gifts that come from awareness that life is not guaranteed and time is limited with the understanding that everything is a choice, life becomes so much richer. I can choose how I react to my situation. I can choose how and with whom I spend my time. I can choose happiness and joy. Because I have a choice, my life is very fulfilling regardless of my health.

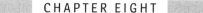 CHAPTER EIGHT

I CONTINUE TO LIVE

OUR WEDDING ANNIVERSARY

Celebrating thirty-five years of marriage was something I wasn't sure would happen when I was diagnosed with lung cancer almost two years ago. So much had transpired on this journey: fear, pain, hope, happiness, inspiration, and more than anything LOVE!

Teresa, my love, I will take however many more days we are gifted together with gratitude and appreciation.

In looking back on these writings, I was surprised to see how prevalent death was in my thoughts. When the doctor said I had a 50% chance of living one year, my life, our lives were turned upside down. While we proceeded with the program to control my cancer, death always lurked as an undercurrent to our thoughts and plans. I had forgotten how this impacted Teresa as well. She was always so calm, attempting to endure the stress without adding to my burden.

Looking back, I could see how tough this had been for her.

Nearly two years later, the journey had become more routine. When we made it past the one-year mark, the thought of death came less frequently. We endured the week after chemo and thrived in the weeks before the next chemo treatment. My philosophy of living each day as if I have three years to live had been liberating in that we could enjoy each day immensely and plan for the near-term future with energy and enthusiasm. I will continue to live each day as a gift. As my doctor told me, "You've already beaten the odds!"

THE UPS AND DOWNS

Before I go on, I want to publicly thank our friends who spent many hours lovingly reviewing all the posts on my blog at CaringBridge, pulling out numerous quotes and pictures, and beautifully putting together a beautiful coffee table book of inspirational posts and reader comments up to the end of 2020. When Teresa and I opened the package, we both cried tears of appreciation, joy, and happiness. Thank you, Jim and Christi.

I would be lying if I said I was never discouraged. At times, the best way to describe my state of mind was despair. I don't know any other word that even comes close to the emotional state I experience in many of the weeks following Healing Friday. By now you know the symptoms and perhaps I am repeating them too often. Welcome to my world!

That week is quite the struggle; both physically and emotionally. My foggy, achy brain made any type of thought challenging. I struggled to put coherent words together while both speaking and writing. I struggled to link thoughts together while attempting to think and I find myself losing concentration and forgetting what I am talking about three words into a sentence. I just feel like a zombie. I get so frustrated I want to cry.

My body feels like I am carrying 400 extra pounds of heaviness inside me. I almost can't believe how difficult it is to move. Even simple things like getting out of my recliner takes an agonizing fifteen to twenty minutes.

I feel listless and useless. I become disgusted with myself.

Thoughts like, *this is not the life I want! The chemo is not worth doing if this is the result, I can't take this anymore, I'm going to quit and let the cards fall where they may* bounce through my brain. All my life I was able to embrace adversity and find ways to work my way through it. I was able to find a mental state that accepted whatever events had occurred and then move on. Sadly, with chemo I often find myself unable to do that.

Pure happiness, however, is not based on circumstance or even physical pain or pleasure. True happiness is a choice. I'm not suggesting it is an easy choice, but a choice it is. Sometimes I struggle to find a reason to be happy during the week after Healing Friday. Whatever happened to me was supposed to happen based on choices I made. When struggling with chemo I thought, *I didn't choose this! I choose not to do this anymore!*

One Saturday, during a good week, Teresa and I were out for a hike. As we were strolling through our local hills, a sudden awareness made me stop in my tracks. I was shocked and welcomed this new thought.

I felt great.

My mind was clear, and I found myself enjoying the beauty around me and the time I was able to spend with my beautiful wife. It was a perfect moment. I found myself thinking, healing week *wasn't so bad! What was the big deal? Chemo resulted in huge emotional swings during every cycle.*

The good times had returned! To take more control of my treatments and create more good times, I planned to push for changes in the chemo strategy at the next meeting with my oncologist. Following are the questions I wanted answered so that we could plan our future:

- What is the long-term impact on me from the intense chemo?
- What are we giving up if we drop the chemo and just do the immunotherapy?
- What if we just cut the chemo in half?
- What options are coming down the road that will be more effective and less debilitating?

A lot of good that did me. The answer to every question I asked was, "it depends."

Around that time, another event happened that made me both grateful and sad. A gentleman who was given the same diagnosis as mine about nine months ago passed away. His family turned to me in the beginning and continued to follow my blog during his cancer journey. I was heartbroken for his family for what they have gone through and must endure. I also felt guilty that I was doing so well. I imagined they were wondering why they couldn't have the quality time that I was enjoying with Teresa, my family, and friends. Since I started this journey, five friends and acquaintances have been diagnosed with cancer and subsequently passed away.

I am acutely aware that my time is limited. I will not squander it.

AND THE BEAT GOES ON

Cancer continued to be a nonevent and chemo continued to be a struggle. Another chemo session resulted in discomfort all the way through the following Saturday. Eight tough days! It seemed that the duration of the discomfort was increasing at a rapid pace.

Near the end of 2020, it was time for another MRI and a CAT scan. They used a process called "with contrast." What this means is they had me drink 24 ounces of radioactive liquid and then filmed me for the CAT scan. After a short filming, they stuck an IV in me and loaded me up with more radiation to create contrast and filmed me again. This process would give a clear picture of any cancerous activity in my entire torso and a good view of my lung tumor. After the scan, they left the IV tube in my arm and sent me over for an MRI. It was a longer process as they rolled me into the MRI cylinder (claustrophobia!) for about fifteen minutes, pulled me out to inject more radioactive fluids into my veins, and then filmed me again for about five minutes (again to create contrast and a better view). The MRI was strictly to look at my brain to ensure that the tumor is gone, and no new tumors had shown up.

To make sure I was as radiant as possible, I went to the dentist after the scan because I lost a crown. The dentist decided I should have an X-ray before he re-glued the crown. Surely, I was glowing all night with all the radioactive materials coursing through me.

Historically, I was excited to have the scans done because I wanted to see how much progress I made with the cancer. For some reason, this particular time I was a little apprehensive. We had nothing but good news on the cancer for 20+ months. For some reason, optimistic Les was wondering when the other shoe would drop, and we would have new spots showing up in the scans. I had done amazingly well so far with no reason for pessimism. But for some reason I couldn't shake it. I've learned that many cancer patients experience the same anxiety with scans asking themselves, "is this the one that will give us the bad news?"

More of the emotional ups and downs from living with cancer!

I've spoken with many survivors of various types of cancer. Most of them were through with chemo in less than half a year. The longest I've heard is eight months. I guess I won the lottery in that I get to do it for the rest of my life. At times, this realization feels like a heavy burden for Teresa and me.

As the meeting with my doctor to go over the results of the scans got closer, more ideas came to mind. We hoped to negotiate a change in treatment after that meeting. I really needed something to change, but not if it meant a high risk of the cancer taking over. I really wanted to push him to think outside the box. I asked him to include the radiation oncologist in our discussions.

The meeting with the doctors arrived and I was excited to hear that they had new plans for me, but first, their comments on progress. The word they used was *stable*. My cancer was stable which, according to Webster's, in a medical sense meant "not getting worse." While I know this is really all we could expect, it is disheartening to hear every time we meet. It is a sobering reminder that my cancer is treatable but not curable.

As usual, we discussed changes in my treatment, the costs, and the benefits. The current treatment was working; I was stable. But at what cost? We could keep the treatment as it was, but over the long haul what other organs would the chemo destroy and how much was my reaction to chemo interfering with my quality of life?

We went over all the ideas I had on how to change up the treatment protocol. We went over how well I was handling the treatments. My oncologist even mentioned that I would soon be his longest continuous patient receiving chemo treatments. The reality is that we should keep going as long as we can with the current chemo treatment until either my cancer evolves/adapts and the treatment stops working, or my body can no longer tolerate chemo. Staying the course appears to be the best option. There may be alternatives down the road, but they are not likely to be more effective.

Before I share our decision about future treatments, I would like to share a behavioral change I employed after my last session. My emotions were heading in the wrong direction once again.

I was allowing the chemo to defeat me.

I didn't know if I could make things better this time by just changing my mindset. At this point in the journey, lifestyle and chemo were at odds. The medicine was controlling more than my cancer and my outlook, it was impacting my life. It was time to change more than how I view my world, I had to change my behavior.

I decided that my reaction to chemo would not get worse if I didn't let it stop me from living. I had to choose to live my life as if I wasn't on chemo and do my best to ignore it.

It may seem odd or "against doctor's order," but I had decided that my active lifestyle and chemo had to start getting along better. On Monday after chemo, I exercised in the morning and worked for a couple of hours. On Tuesday after chemo, I was defeated and rested all day. On Wednesday after chemo, I exercised in the morning, lead a group meeting, and had two one-to-one meetings. On Thursday after chemo, I had a morning meeting and played a round of golf. I felt so much better than if I had allowed the process to continue controlling me. I wasn't forcing these two to play nice, mind you. Chemo wins the day of and most days after treatment, but as soon as I was able, activity started in earnest.

Was I uncomfortable?

Yes.

Now, our decision on future treatments...

We decided to cut the chemo component of my treatment by 1/3 and leave the immunotherapy untouched. Hopefully, this small change would make the recovery from Healing Friday more palatable while continuing to hold the cancer at bay. It was a risk, but one we chose to take. My doctor seemed happy with our decision; however, he seemed more concerned with ensuring the quality of my life than he was about extending my life. Teresa and I would prefer to achieve both!

Whenever I met with the doctor, I was reminded that I was living on borrowed time. They seemed to relish using the word "incurable" when discussing my cancer. I found myself asking lots of questions about how best to use the time I had left, whether it was one year, three years, or ten years. The good news was I had many options. The bad news was that I had many options, and I couldn't do them all. COVID wasn't helping.

How did the reduced chemo work after the last treatment?

The experiment was a wash. The first days after chemo were pretty much as tough as they always had been. In fact, the following Monday might have been my toughest Monday yet.

> *I want to encourage all of you to make the most of every day, find joy in each other, and love fully. I have no regrets in my life, please don't let yourselves have any regrets either.*

However, by Wednesday I was starting to feel pretty good and was pretty much back to normal by Friday. The real test would be how I handled the next treatment. I was hoping there would be a reverse cumulative effect and I would feel better by Tuesday. Unfortunately, I was disappointed since there was no change in my reaction for months thereafter.

The October meeting clarified for me just how serious they considered my condition to be. My oncologist made it clear that he was both pleased and surprised that I was still around. For the first time, he admitted that once lung cancer metastasizes in the brain, the clock starts ticking and, in his experience, the window is six to twelve months. I've known this was true but he had never come out and said it until now.

People with serious diseases like mine just don't last long.

Alex Trebek is an example of a person diagnosed with cancer (not the same as mine) who passed away in less than one year. This had me thinking about how near to death I might be and how amazingly fortunate I continued to be that my results were *stable*. My oncologist continued to focus on strategies to "make me comfortable and allow me to enjoy the time I have left."

The brain surgeon was another story! First, he was blunt in a refreshing way. He always called my cancer "incurable lung cancer." He appeared very surprised that I was still around and believed that I might be a case that rewrites all the rules. He wanted to "think outside the box" and start treating my cancer as if it were stage III rather than stage IV.

What that meant was that he wanted to put me into a radiation treatment designed to destroy the tumors in my lungs and two lymph nodes. This is a common approach to several cancers that have not migrated to other parts of the body and are therefore stage I, II, or III. His belief was that since the little cancer cells running through my blood stream had not found a new host to attack, we could kill the big boys so that they couldn't mutate and trust that the chemo treatments would continue to keep the little boys at bay for a few years longer. I think he saw the potential to write an article about my success if this procedure bought me five or more extra years. We all agreed to this strategy.

NEW STRATEGY, MORE TESTS

The first thing we had to do was a new PET scan to make sure everything looked good for this process. Next, my primary oncologist, who was not committed, and I had to agree on this path (Teresa and I were 100% committed). Then we would start six weeks of radiation therapy where I would go in every day, Monday through Friday, for targeted radiation. The chemo treatments would continue as well during this process. At the end, hopefully, there would be no active tumors. Nothing would likely change with my chemo schedule afterwards. We didn't discuss side effects of radiation which would become a major issue down the road.

All this talk and effort had me thinking again about how inevitable death was for me in the near term (who knew how near). I thought about it a lot, especially how I wanted to spend the time I had left. I remained disgusted that COVID was putting a damper on how I/we enjoyed our days. I was hopeful that Teresa and I could be early recipients of a vaccine so that we could get out with friends more comfortably, travel more safely, and enjoy our lives.

Little did we know the many mutations of COVID would linger for years.

My situation had me much less impacted by the goings on in the world. I found myself living more in the moment. The past was the past and there was absolutely nothing I could change. The future wouldn't exist until I got there. It seemed that I could only live in the present and if I was true to myself, my beliefs, and values and genuinely cared about others in my life, then I couldn't go wrong by living each day filled with love, gratitude, and appreciation. I couldn't believe how joyful my life was as I lived in this peaceful place with the woman of my dreams.

We started the radiation phase of my treatment in early December 2020. I was "mapped" for the radiation treatment and little alignment dots were tattooed to my chest. I was not 100% sure what the treatment entailed or how it would affect me. What I did know was that I had to go in for treatment every weekday for six+ weeks. The actual timing would be shared with me at my session on December eighth. Apparently, most people don't have anything else in their lives but cancer treatment, so the doctors don't worry too much about scheduling conflicts.

Perhaps I needed to focus more on my treatment than on other aspects of my life...

Nah, I liked how it was going.

It was ironic that I started feeling anxious and melancholy after my "mapping" appointment. Somehow the change in treatment was causing me to think more about my cancer journey. This was a big move.

- Would it make a difference?
- What would the treatments be like for me?
- How would six weeks of treatment impact the rest of my activities?
- How would my Vistage members handle me being gone for six weeks?
- How could I live out my remaining days?
- What changes should I be considering?

Funny, just writing this down in my blog relieved my anxiety. This was such an amazing life and death adventure.

I was surprised at how little fear and despair had shown up for me. After two years of chemo, I was confident I was not in denial, so why did so many days feel like just another day in my life? Having incurable lung cancer was part of who I was but it didn't define or change my core self. Sometimes, I wondered if I was human based on how I responded to having cancer. I even asked myself, *what is wrong with me?* Sure, I had moments, but they didn't last, and they didn't change my outlook. I was grateful for the way I was; I just wanted to understand how I became this way.

RADIATION

I started radiation in early December and got it every weekday except Christmas and New Year's. Radiation was scheduled to end on January 22. The radiation experience was essentially a non-event. I showed up, took off my shirt, laid down on a table, and had two radiation technicians adjust my body using laser indicators and my new tattoo dots. Then they zapped me with radiation for a couple of minutes. The whole process took about ten minutes and I felt nothing. When I left, I felt a sunburn-like tightness on my chest, and I had an intermittent cough.

If only that was the end of it. After three weeks of radiation, it was really starting to kick my butt. First and foremost was the fatigue. I have run ten marathons, bicycled from Oregon to San Diego, and walked 500 miles across Spain. I've climbed to the top of mount Whitney and the bottom of the Grand Canyon, and I had never felt fatigue like the kind I got after radiation. My entire body was exhausted. I struggled to even write or play my ukulele. Even reading was challenging. It was such a departure from my normal high energy state that I found myself disoriented and discombobulated. It is hard to fathom how a few moments of radiation could tear me down so much.

I was so glad that I chose to start a sabbatical from work during radiation because I didn't believe I could have been effective.

Thank you, Fred Chaney, for leading my groups during my absence.

Fatigue soon became the least of my concerns. I had trouble swallowing or even drinking. It felt as if there was a blockage in my esophagus. Everything, including dry swallowing, felt as if a ball of needles was slowly working its way down my throat. Add to this the occasional, sudden, painful cramping in my esophagus that strikes for about thirty seconds and makes the overall experience miserable, and you can imagine the extent of the pain.

By now, you realize I had a core belief that if I stopped doing things, I would start the process of dying. I've seen too many people that choose to slow down when sick or in pain "until they feel better" and never come back. Usually, something else would pop up and they slow down some more. I refused to let that happen to me, so I continued to exercise every day. I continued to play progressively poorer golf, and I continued to be a friend and mentor to those who wanted me. Santa even brought Teresa and me e-bikes so that we could get out even more in the days to come. My promise to myself, to Teresa, and to all who cared was that I would keep moving forward until I absolutely could not function, period!

It hurt me to see the pain on Teresa's face as she watched me struggle. I knew that she felt helpless. I knew that she hurt as much for me as I hurt. I greatly appreciated the empathy; I just wished I could do something to make it easier on her. She was sacrificing constantly to stay by my side throughout this experience. It was just one more reason I loved her more and more every day.

TESTIMONIAL: SCOTT VON LUFT

I met Scott through Vistage. He was younger than me and was just starting out on his leadership journey. Here is what Scott had to say:

I was connected to Les by a mutual acquaintance, someone who used to be in Les's other CEO group. I was going to be taking over a new position and thought, hey, this could be a good experience. I had two Vistage chairs that I met with, and we were interviewing each other. I connected well with Les and said, "You've got to be my Vistage chair."

I didn't believe in myself at all. And I had a lot of doubts as to whether to take the position and whether I would have the courage to do it. Beyond that, I needed to be everything, do everything, and I had to be the best, smartest person. Otherwise, I was an ineffective CEO. He helped change some of my thinking and throw out the head trash.

The biggest aha moment for me was that Les spent the first year working with me trying to get my head clear. It took a year before I could really be effective in my role because I was just getting run over left and right. I remember I would call him on occasion, just like an emotional mess. And he said, "Well, Scott, let's start using knowledge and skills that we've been developing for the last few weeks. You got it, now you just need to start doing it." And it was like a lightbulb moment for me, I thought maybe I can start implementing some of the stuff that we had been talking about.

Les really tried to instill in me that my role is more about who I am and less about what I do. It was more about how I show up and support others rather than "you're the one in charge." I had it in my head that that I had to be in charge.

He said, "One day, you're gonna wake up and you're going to be in charge, you don't need to go around telling everyone that you're in charge." That was the aha moment where I could lay down the battle axe and stop fighting against my people.

And I learned to talk about the direction of vision, to get my employees involved rather than telling them. A lot of people that I was being asked to lead had seen me in lesser roles, and you know, younger in my life. I was trying to go from being on the team or even working for some of the people on the leadership team to now leading the team. He helped me with that and helped me develop the patience I needed to be effective.

He said, "Just give it time and get some wins, and you'll just be in charge, you don't have to say I'm in charge." It was very good advice. When I found out the guy's got incurable cancer, it helped me refocus on what my life was about and what I was doing.

I lost my dad when I was young. And Les filled that void, giving me encouragement when I needed it. When he got diagnosed, I was like, oh, shit, we're going through this again. How it changed for me was I became even more committed to not being the one that had to do everything. I figured out that we need to build an organization that can run without us, because at any moment, our stories can change. And there are so many people that are reliant and dependent on what it is *that we're doing. Because of that, we can't hold it in. We must share with everybody so that our purpose can survive.*

I'm not a religious guy by any means. But I feel like Les has functioned as a guardian angel for me. I love it. He helped to get my head straight. He's been a source of wisdom and leadership. And through this process, dealing with this cancer, he's really showing and leading us all like this is how you deal with cancer.

LESSONS LEARNED: DEATH IS NOT A FOUR-LETTER WORD

People often told me they were impressed with my mindset and the "one step at a time" attitude I had. I was glad I could be this way. That said, mortality does cross my mind at times during the day. We are all going to die someday, we just don't know when. My time could be thirty years from now or next year. Whenever it happens, it will be cancer related. What I am taken by is the cognitive bias known as the *Frequency Illusion* or the Baader-Meinhof effect. Since being diagnosed with cancer, I saw articles, heard stories, read headlines, and experienced news reports about people dying from cancer every day. This awareness didn't elude me, and it wouldn't define me either. But, for brief moments I allowed myself to wonder, *Is this it? Are we on a no-win path?* They are fleeting moments, but don't assume I was immune from having them.

I lived my life intentionally for the past fifteen years with the personal mission statement, "help others achieve the greatness within them." I was blessed to be successful in this mission in many ways throughout the years and I intend for my journey to help others endure and thrive in their similar journeys. This gives me great peace as we walk this road of uncertain distance. I will continue to strive to be a beacon of hope and a conduit to personal greatness for those I am fortunate enough to touch in my life.

Most of you know I am not a religious person. I do believe there is an energy or a force that unites all of us. I can feel it now more than ever. The prayers of loved ones embraced me every moment of every day. I could truly feel it. Knowing that I have Buddhist, Hindu, Muslim, Sikh, Jewish, and Christian prayers coming my way gives me so much strength.

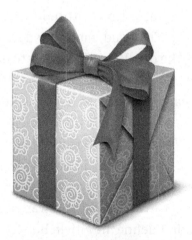

THE GIFT OF POSSIBILITIES

Most of this book you hold in your hands is about my life, my lifestyle, living, and hopefully, some lessons and values you can embrace in your life. While the story of my journey may be detailed, it's important to read between the lines as you finish this book. Notice that I seldom dwell on what I "can't" do and focus my thoughts and energy on what I "can" do.

Death, in my opinion, is not to be feared. Death is not to be embraced, either. Living, as it turns out is simple a journey where each day, moment, and second is precious. Our minds often drift to the past and future. With an imminent death, life becomes more vibrant, and you feel more alive.

Cancer has placed many obstacles in my path that in the moment are more real than my eventual death. I can't do as much as I once did, work is a challenge, my ukulele skills have not returned, I've lost much of my physicality, and on and on. Yet, I don't let any of this get me down or stop me.

I focus on what is possible!

Possibility is such a gift for me. When I see there is something difficult in my path, I ask myself what can I do? If I cannot finger pick a song, I choose to strum it and sing along. If I cannot surf, I paddle out and hang out with the other surfers. If I cannot ride a bike up a mountain, I ride an e-bike. If there is an obstacle placed in front of me by cancer or life in general, I put zero energy into wishing it wasn't there and all my energy into identifying what is possible.

I have often said that when a person claims they can't do something, they are stepping into a self-limiting belief. They are holding onto a belief masquerading as a fact. Whenever you hear yourself saying, "I can't do that." Ask yourself, "what can I do?" Focus on what is possible and let go of believing obstacles block your path to happiness and enjoyment.

The world is full of possibilities for all of us. Find what is possible and do it!

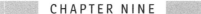 CHAPTER NINE

RADIATION SIDE EFFECTS

Because of the radiation, I was in pain all the time. It was not severe pain, maybe a two on a scale of one to ten, but it was constant. The pain was like a stiffening in my chest and upper back. About twice an hour, it spasmed to a more severe cramp. The worst part was eating. When I ate, the pain jumped up to an eight throughout the meal. The doctor gave me a prescription to help with the pain, but I found that it only worked *after* I ate. If I drink it before I eat, the effect stopped about halfway through the meal.

I was tired all the time, lacked ambition, and ran out of gas quickly. I felt as if another person had invaded my body. As someone who has taken pride in his energy and endurance, I felt diminished and a little less than human. Throughout my life I've observed so many couples where the wife takes care of the husband in their later years, and I have tremendous fear that will happen to me/us. I knew that Teresa would be fine with taking care of me, I just didn't want to become a burden as my cancer progressed.

When I discussed the pain with my radiation oncologist, he dropped a bit of a bombshell on me that I am sure I/we had not heard before. I asked him what the radiation was going to do for the long term. His response was, "The last scan showed that the tumor had grown a little, therefore the chemo is not working as well on the tumor. Radiation will allow us to eliminate that tumor and let the chemo take care of preventing/delaying future tumors." We had no idea that the tumor had grown. It was a reminder to me that we were just buying time with the chemo and eventually new tumors would show up.

The side effects of radiation compounded my lost ability to envision a future.

I spent my entire life thinking about and planning five to ten years in the future. I always believed that if I could envision something, I could make it happen. I just had to decide who I wanted to be, what I needed to do, and what I had to have to achieve that future and then make it happen. Through cancer treatments and now radiation I was losing my ability to dream and that was very sad for me.

More negativity was flowing into my brain.

GLAD RADIATION IS BEHIND US

I finished radiation on January 21, 2021, and then had chemo the next day. I was finally back physically and mentally. I was surprised that the pain from radiation increased after we stopped zapping my lungs. Apparently, my body was protecting me from the pain during the daily doses and then once that stopped, my body focused more on healing than pain control. We would not know for a month or two if we got all the lung cancer. We were waiting until the inflammation caused by radiation diminished so that we could get an accurate reading.

I took a two-month sabbatical from work during radiation. Traditionally, sabbaticals are designed to allow a person to rest their mind and rejuvenate. That didn't work for me. There really was no relief from cancer, radiation, nor struggles in life. I remained positive and upbeat, but I could tell that I was not mentally and emotionally the person I've always been. Foolishly, I returned to searching for more information about longevity with my type of cancer. I already knew the five-year survival rate was 5%. I learned that there are two types of stage IV lung cancer. Stage 4a (spreads in chest area) has a five-year survival rate of 5%, and stage 4b (spreads beyond chest area, i.e., brain) has a five-year survival rate of less than 1%. I guessed that was why the doctors were so surprised when they saw me. I was an aberration.

What did this knowledge do to me mentally and emotionally?

I felt as if I was walking down a dark alley with no end in sight. In fact, I was destined never to find my way out of the alley. I was being stalked by an unseen assailant who I could sense but not see or hear. I knew it was there. I could feel it. I was anticipating it striking out at me, but I couldn't tell when or where. I was constantly on edge, wondering and waiting. I was tense and filled with stress. I could feel it changing me, changing how I showed up.

I needed to find a way to ease the burden. I needed to make changes; I just didn't know what changes. Teresa and I were talking about our future, and we would continue to do so. The next years of my life will be full, we just need to determine what they will be filled with. I promised Teresa ten more years from the day I was diagnosed (she keeps moving the bar by saying that's ten years from today, every day). I live with the thought that I have three years to live from each day. Can you imagine what it is like to live your life where everyday thoughts of how long you are going to live, wondering how many times you will get to do what you are doing, and are you going to be able to do what you dream of doing sits in the back of your mind?

> *Please don't worry about me, I really am in high spirits. I just think it is important to share the emotional toll this crazy situation is taking on me. I believe my optimism and love of life gives me a leg up on other people in a similar situation. Every person who sees me is shocked that I have not changed in appearance at all. I remain full of life, joy, and happiness.*

Teresa and I were sitting in the airport lounge awaiting our first flight to Hawaii since COVID. I was finally traveling again after a year in COVID purgatory. We received our first vaccine, we tested negative, and we felt safe and secure traveling again.

It was eleven weeks since the start of radiation and four weeks since completion. I was finally starting to feel like my old self. My energy was coming back slowly; the pain and discomfort was almost gone. (It was still painful to eat and drink, however.) And my spirits were back to their normal high level. Looking back, I was surprised at how radiation impacted me emotionally. I felt down and defeated, and it showed up in my everyday activities and perspectives. I could see it much more clearly after it was all over than I did when I was in it. It felt good to be me again.

February was one of the most emotionally fulfilling months of my life. It was my birthday month (I would be 66 on the 24th). A group of past and current members/clients got together and decided that each day one of them would send me a note or video sharing with me how something I did or said impacted their lives well beyond business. Some of these people I hadn't seen in five years, yet they took the time to share their stories. I was humbled and proud. I shed tears of joy every time I received one of these messages. What a special gift these wonderful people gave me!

Did the radiation do its job?

We were waiting for my body to heal fully from the radiation before doing my next scans in mid-April. I had doctors' appointments scheduled for the first week of May to review those scans and check the status of my tumor and lymph nodes. I focused on enjoying and maximizing every day.

THE STOCKDALE PARADOX

I often wonder why I seem to handle my diagnosis better than many others. I might have come up with an answer. During a workshop with my members, we discussed the Stockdale Paradox. Admiral Stockdale was a prisoner of war in Vietnam. He shared that the prisoners who hoped they would be released by Christmas, and then Valentine's

Day, and then Easter, and so on were always disappointed and disheartened and suffered much worse than those who accepted the fact that they were going to be there a long time. Those who didn't put a date on their eventual release still had hope that they would be going home, they just didn't set themselves up for disappointment.

I accepted that at some point in the future, cancer would kill me. I was in no hurry to have that happen and I intended to live every day to the fullest. What I refused to do is use words like, I am "battling" cancer, I am a "survivor," or we are going to win this "fight." That mindset could only lead to disappointments after every set back. I would be depressed if I looked at my cough or fatigue as a lost battle. My mindset was that I was thriving with cancer regardless of the situations it placed in front of me. If I needed to adjust, I could and would.

THE GREAT MISTAKE — OR THE MEDICAL PROFESSION ISN'T PERFECT

The results of my blood test on March 25, 2021 showed that my thyroid numbers were out of whack. When I showed up for chemo the next morning, I was told that I had a prescription for thyroid medicine waiting for me in the pharmacy. I really didn't know what an out of whack thyroid meant. I did know that it was a common side effect of chemo so it could just be that the chemo had started to degrade my thyroid gland. The less attractive alternative was that cancer has found its way into the thyroid.

Chemo fatigue was a huge issue ...again.

I struggled to keep my eyes open throughout the day. On several occasions, I found myself falling asleep at unexpected times. It seemed as if my chemo side effects were more excessive. Was it the thyroid?

A new development was a pronounced cough. It was especially present after minor exertion. The cough seemed to last about five minutes then went away until the next outbreak. My guess was that this was a product of the scar tissue from the radiation breaking down or possibly it was an expansion of the lung cancer. It had Teresa concerned.

We scheduled a CAT scan and an MRI for April 22. I would meet with the doctor the beginning of May to find out what was really going on inside of me. I asked him what would happen if the radiation didn't work and the treatments stopped working. He said we would try something new but as a rule those new choices are less effective than the course we were on.

The thyroid medicine was causing me all sorts of issues. I sat down to write a note to my doctor to share all the side effects I was getting from the thyroid medicine. I went back to my medical records to check the numbers so that I could be accurate in my communication. *When I looked, it showed my thyroid numbers as normal!?!* There was a note under the test results that said, "We did a quality check on your numbers and a mistake was made, these are the correct numbers." This happened a day after the initial numbers were posted but they did not inform me nor my doctor.

I shared this discovery with my doctor along with listing the side effects. To say the least, he was livid that nobody told him. Effective immediately, we stopped the thyroid medication. The next day, I felt great! Things went back to status quo as your everyday stage IV cancer patient with chemo-related side effects.

HARD TIMES, MAY 2021

It was a tough four weeks. My breathing became difficult. If I tried to walk and talk or climb a flight of stairs, my airway became completely blocked. The cough was intense. I came close to going to the emergency room one evening because I couldn't seem to get a full breath.

What was happening to my lungs?

As usual, I did not allow the breathing issue to get in the way of living. Teresa and I went up to Monterey to enjoy the beauty and play a few rounds of golf. I sent a note to my doctor while we were up there explaining the severity of my breathing situation and his nurse/assistant called me while I was playing golf at Spyglass Hill. They wanted to set me up with an appointment for the next day, but I had plans to play Pebble Beach so I told them I couldn't get back for the appointment. We decided to wait until my scheduled meeting with the doctor on May 10.

Interestingly, we were paired up with an oncologist at Spyglass. The oncologist saw my stressful breathing, and when I explained that I had lung cancer and just had radiation he said, "Oh, you have radiation pneumonitis. It is common with lung radiation and can be resolved with a steroid."

That sounded like pneumonia to me.

The next day, I received the write up on my CT scan and the analyst wrote that he could not see the results of the radiation on my tumor because the image was obscured by "acute radiation pneumonitis" thus confirming my playing partner's diagnosis. Unfortunately, I had not met with or spoken to my doctor, so I had no prescription for a steroid that I assumed was an inhaler. I did find an over-the-counter inhaler that would give relief. Teresa had to visit seven pharmacies to track one down! The relief was instant though temporary, but I counted it as a win.

My life would have been so much easier if I had known that radiation pneumonitis was a possible side effect.

The analyst of the CT scan could see the part of the lung not obscured by pneumonitis and identified three new spots. That was concerning. We would not allow ourselves to be too concerned until we talked to the oncologist, however. Perhaps there would be changes in my program, perhaps not. I was getting a little complacent, believing the chemo was working so well at keeping the cancer at bay. While the information was not unexpected, it was a bummer.

A few weeks later, we met with the doctor, and it turned out that the three spots seen on the last scan were not cancer. The doctor thought it might be more of the radiation pneumonitis that plagued me since January. As to the pneumonitis, I went into the doctor's office about two weeks before my planned appointment and just sat there until they took care of me. They took an X-ray to confirm the diagnosis and then put me on mega doses of prednisone pills. It took a while, but the prednisone finally started working, and I was able to breathe freely.

The oncologist also took me off of Keytruda because he believed Keytruda was exacerbating my breathing issues. This really had me scared because I believed Keytruda was the drug keeping me alive.

In mid-year 2021 I wrote, "This two-and-a-half-year journey took more of a toll on me than I realized, especially with the challenges of the past five months. I hadn't realized the impact the stress of chemo every three weeks, the one week of sickness each time, the desire to be present and effective in my work, and the desire to be present for family and friends was placing on my psychological state. I found myself waking up angry and frustrated that I had to continue struggling to push through. Something had to change!"

I announced my retirement from work.

I dreamed of doing this work well into my 80s. I loved the impact I had on amazing people who had an even greater impact on so many others. I made a difference in many people's lives and that was a beautiful thing. Unfortunately, I had to admit that I just couldn't keep it up. Being sick seventeen weeks out of the year and trying to act like nothing was happening just wouldn't cut it. The past few months had me wondering if this was my last year of my life. I found myself reluctant to make plans beyond a few months out. I saw the end and wanted to make sure I was prepared for it. There was a lot going on in my head. It was time.

We met with the doctor, and I reminded him that Teresa was expecting me to live ten more years from today. He said that was a big ask but he was up for the challenge. He also said he was excited about the many changes in cancer treatments that were coming down the road. He really sounded optimistic which was nice for a change.

THE PREDNISONE DEBACLE

I was on a continuous downward spiral. It all started with the radiation and then just continued its downward trajectory from there. I was having trouble breathing, and I couldn't speak or walk without coughing. I would even cough about every sixty seconds while sitting. Looking back, I believe I went into a state of depression. I had been on prednisone for about two weeks.

Prednisone is a powerful steroid intended to eliminate the inflammation that was making it so hard to breath. After taking mega doses of prednisone (80 mg) for a little over two weeks, we went through a 3+ week step down process to wean me off the drug.

The entire prednisone experience was debilitating. First, the side effects were normally hyperactivity and weight gain. For me, the side effects were lethargy and weight loss. I lost ten lbs. in four weeks and found myself unmotivated and exhausted. I couldn't get myself to write, to play the ukulele, or to even read. Whatever I tried seemed like too much work. If I was sitting on the couch, I had to psych myself up to go to the bathroom or to get a drink of water. Everything felt like a major effort. Walking up a flight a stairs took great effort. If Teresa wanted to go somewhere, I was worried about how far I would have to walk.

The low point came when I went out to Scottsdale with a group of friends to play golf (a trip that had been planned months in advance). With the heat at 100 degrees, I was destroyed. I couldn't play golf at all. I just sat in the cart with cold towels on me until someone took me to my room to sleep and cool off. The next day was cooler but more of the same. I was constantly on the verge of passing out.

I was in desperate need of a win.

We spoke to the doctor when I returned from Arizona, and he indicated that he was not surprised by how I was reacting. He said it could take up to a year for my body to completely recover from the radiation and several months for my body to recover from the prednisone. He also informed me that the prednisone would not cure the pneumonitis, it would just get my body on the right track for recovery. It could take a few more months to end the pneumonitis. While I was disappointed that nobody told me this before I started, I probably would not have changed my decision to proceed with the radiation and the prednisone.

On the positive side, things began looking up after returning home. I was able to go to the gym. I gained back 2 lbs. I felt like playing the ukulele again. I only coughed when I exerted myself or tried to sing. I was even able to write a blog post which felt like a major challenge just a few days prior. I knew that things would get better, it was just going to take a little longer than I had hoped.

We still seemed to have the cancer under control. Funny, I hadn't thought about cancer for a while. I wondered what it meant when the cure and repair from the cure were more important than the disease.

The bottom line was that I've had a relatively easy go of it in my cancer journey though you might not believe it reading this book. Most people had a much tougher time. Although the first six months in 2021 were awful, I knew that my cancer remained under control and that my future looked bright. Every day I felt a little stronger, I was breathing a little better, and seeing the world a little brighter. I was looking forward to tomorrow and all the tomorrows after that.

FEELING GREAT! FALL 2021

I was feeling better than I had felt since before radiation. I felt strong, I gained back my weight, I was breathing freely even during exercise, and my mind was clear. I had forgotten what it was like to feel so good.

What changed? I was finally over the effects of the prednisone and the radiation. Also, another plug for advocating for myself. I spoke to the doctor and shared that I had lived with exercise induced asthma for the first forty years of my life. I carried an inhaler around with me that I used prior to intense workouts and in case of a breathing emergency. I asked him if he could prescribe the same inhaler for my current state.

"Umm, I never really thought about that, let me look up what's available," he mumbled. "Oh, that's interesting," he exclaimed, "here's a steroid-based inhaler that you take twice a day that just might do the trick. I'll prescribe it and the asthma inhaler you requested, and we will see what happens."

I began using the inhaler twice a day and within two days, I was breathing better. Four weeks later, I was breathing as well as ever. It surprised me that the doctor was not aware of this option since I've been told that 40% of lung cancer patients who get radiation get pneumonitis. Again, this proved that, when dealing with our health, we must advocate for ourselves and do the research ourselves. Doctors are awesome, just not perfect, and they do not know everything.

A few months later, I had another tough bout with vertigo. My head was spinning for six hours. It was disconcerting. It finally stopped when I went in for my 90-minute lymphatic massage (my first lymphatic massage since COVID-19 happened; I forgot how much they can hurt).

We performed another CT scan of my body and MRI of my brain, and both were analyzed as unremarkable. Isn't that amazing? What "unremarkable" meant was that there were no active tumors anywhere in my body, only scar tissue from the tumors that had been destroyed. I wonder if that was the first time somebody had called me unremarkable.

Unfortunately, I continued to see my strength and endurance diminish as time went by. It seemed the cancer had cut into my lung capacity even though it wasn't expanding. I had trouble keeping up with the others while my expectation was that I would be leading the pack. A big part of it was the radiation pneumonitis which continued to afflict me. The doctor expected me to be dealing with that for months.

Teresa and I were fortunate to be cruising the Adriatic with thirty friends on a private yacht, the *Black Swan*. We departed Split and bounced around the islands enjoying great food, great sights, and great friendship. We were ecstatic to be traveling again. I also felt bulletproof after receiving my third COVID shot. For a brief period, I felt normal. Even the words cancer and chemo had not entered my brain for a day or so. I felt so good, when the ship stopped and everyone decided to dive into the ocean, I jumped right in and started swimming. About 100 yards from the ship, my brain reminded me of my condition. "Hey Les, don't forget you have incurable cancer and are in radiation and chemotherapy," my body reminded me in a profound way.

As I turned and swam out about 100 yards from the ship, I discovered I could not breathe.

No air was getting to my lungs, and I was all alone. I quickly stopped swimming and rolled onto my back as I calmed myself for a few moments. As I turned to make my way back to the ship, a few noticed my despair and brought me swimming noodles. Teresa ran to our berth to fetch my emergency albuterol. After a quick inhale of this miracle elixir, I was good as new.

Lesson learned: take a hit off of the albuterol before swimming. Another lesson: don't be the tough guy, and make sure I have people with me regardless of how easy I feel the task is.

LEGACY

My thoughts begin to hyper-focus on legacy as I walk hand in hand on this journey with Teresa. If I can accomplish anything in the years I have left, whether it be the ten years I promise to Teresa every morning, three years I committed to myself at the beginning of this journey, or even the year I have left on the initial prognosis, it will be to make the path easier, less frightening, and more loving for those who are walking with me, and those who follow me on my path...a Camino de cancer.

Who knows what the future will bring as Teresa and I move forward on this journey?

> *"A heart is not judged by how much you love, but by how much you are loved by others."*
> —**The Wizard of Oz to the Tin Man**

I continued to handle my cancer and the chemo regimen easily. At one point, I felt a slight pain just under my right rib cage that had my attention. *Is the cancer growing in my lung?* I was supposed to see the doctor Monday (11/29/21) but he had a major car accident and he had to cancel. I was trying to navigate the appointment labyrinth to set up a new appointment. They certainly didn't make it easy! When I finally got to see another oncologist during my doctor's absence, he started by saying, "I am surprised you are here, I would not have expected you to live this long." Rather than be uplifted by this comment, my mind went to, "oh darn, I wonder when the cancer will realize it should be killing me."

An active mind might not always be my friend.

I had been off Keytruda for about five months and wanted to get back to having that as part of my program. You may recall, my doctor temporarily cancelled the Keytruda because he felt it was exacerbating the breathing problems I was having post radiation. I had been breathing freely for three months so I felt it was time. His response was that we were doing fine without it, and he wanted to save it for when the tumor grew or new tumors showed up, and we needed a new strategy. I was not sure I understood his logic but went with it anyway.

I was thinking about how cancer impacted me every single day. The obvious scenarios revolved around scheduling activities before, during, and after my healing week. In addition, my first reaction to every little pain was, "is this a tumor?" I didn't really get anxious, it was just that cancer was the first thing to cross my mind. If you pay attention, you would be surprised to see how many times in a week you feel little twinges, phantom pains, and real pains. Imagine how you would feel if your first reaction was always, "is this it? Has the cancer started to attack the rest of my body?"

Always, always, always in the back of my mind was the concern, "when is this going to get bad?" Knowing that my cancer was "incurable" and that it would eventually attack other parts of my body was a constant reminder of my precarious situation. Every person I met that I hadn't seen in months or years was stunned by how healthy I looked and how vibrant I acted. The shock I saw on their faces was also a reminder of my situation.

People in and around my life continued to be afflicted with cancer and their symptoms were much more impactful and debilitating than mine. My cousin's husband informed me that he had cancer. He was going in for a biopsy to determine what type of cancer he had so that they could provide the most targeted therapy possible. He had been in pain for months, he lost 50 lbs., and he struggled to sleep. I kept asking myself, "why is this so easy for me when it is so miserable for people I love?"

His reaction to his diagnosis reminded me of the mental process I went through and other cancer patients have shared with me. The first thing we all experienced was disbelief: "this can't be happening to me, there must be a mistake!" Or "the next test will show that it's really not that bad." I find it is a great challenge for our minds to wrap around the word CANCER. It's even harder when the words terminal or incurable are added to it.

I am sorry to say that his cancer was too far along, and he passed away a few months after diagnosis.

I found myself looking at all the people who smoked and did not have lung cancer. I would see them and think, "why the heck do I have lung cancer while you are standing there puffing on what is probably your 20th cigarette of the day?" Here I was judging people because I was sick and resentful. Then I fell into varying degrees of depression, thinking that my life would end soon.

Trying to determine how to say goodbye to those I love was the most painful aspect of it all. How could I communicate my gratitude and appreciation for all the people who had supported, influenced, mentored, and believed in me throughout my life? How could I make sure that Teresa had a good life after I was gone?

And finally, there was acceptance. Everybody with incurable cancer gets to the point of accepting that this is their/our life. We needed to make choices that reflect a much shorter runway. I will finish with a thought that sits in my little head whenever I see family and friends battling cancer or the courageous people sitting in the oncology department.

I constantly ask myself:

- Why is this so easy for me and so hard for most others?
- Should I hide how well I am doing, or should I continue to act like my situation is possible for them?
- Is it fair that I am thriving while so many others are struggling?
- Am I making too big a deal about my cancer when others have it so much worse?

TESTIMONIAL: SUSAN SMITH

I met Susan Smith through Vistage. She was another tenured chair and a person I considered my close friend. In her own words:

I'm a fellow Vistage chair. In fact, we both became chair emeritus the same year. I don't remember exactly where I met Les. But I do remember enjoying his company at the Boulder, Colorado Keepers of the Flame. That's an event that tenure chairs go to on a yearly basis. I attended every international conference, and he was usually there.

I remember the day that he got the phone call with his doctors saying that he had lung cancer. There were about eight of us sitting around a table and he got up to take the phone call.

He said, "I have to take this call because it's my doctor."

So, he left the table. When he came back and told us, he just looked like he was in a state of shock. As I recall, Linda Hughes, another chair from California, offered to drive him home.

Afterwards, he started to keep the Caring Bridge journal. And it was so impactful. I looked forward to hearing from him. And when he would go an extra week or two without posting, I got concerned.

I am inspired by his persistence and his perseverance and his courage and his positive attitude. I mean, one of the greatest assets he has physically is his smile. One time, I was working out with him. We just happened to both be down at the gym at the same time. And I took a picture of the two of us there. I remember showing it to some of my friends and saying, this was a friend of mine who just got hit with this big bad news and he didn't even look sick.

I met Teresa for the first time, and I felt like I knew her a little bit just from Facebook posts and from everything that he wrote. I always admire men who speak so highly of their wives with such love and respect. He talked about how sorry he was that he was going to be leaving her and that she would have to deal with missing him. I think it showed a lot of sensitivity. He is the one dying, but his focus is on his wife.

Another thing I really admire about him is that he can just plow through the hard times. The Healing Friday (as he calls it) and the ten days afterwards where he is sick, he says he feels fine, like he doesn't even have cancer.

In one of his journal entries, he talked about a meeting where he laid in the back of the room and slept. And I think he might have started snoring or something. And he said his group was just so supportive of him. But the fact that he would go to a meeting, I was shocked at how long he continued to chair.

I talk about him a lot, too, in terms of sharing what he's going through. And, you know, I'm proud that I know him. I was at a Vistage chair group where they mentioned that he was getting this perseverance award. The Regional Vice President said, "How many of you know Les?" I was proud to put my hand up.

I think about him often. If that happens to me, I'll use him as an example of how to handle it, and how to fight it. He's a model for, you know, transparency and expressiveness. And it's not uncommon with Vistage chairs. So, it's nice to see how solid he is in that tradition. He is learning about himself, and yet willing to share it with others and be transparent about what's going on both good and bad. That's an inspiring model for me to know the power of being vulnerable.

It was great to see him at the conference this past summer in Las Vegas. He looked great. He had a big smile on his face most the time. It was the midst of COVID, so it was kind of hard to not hug him. I think he was hugging a lot of people that weekend.

LESSONS LEARNED: DO IT NOW... WHATEVER IT IS

There is no excuse to put off whatever it is that will bring you and those around you joy. Unless your to-do list includes robbing a bank or some other criminal act, all the reasons you can think of for not living your life fully and joyfully are just stories we tell ourselves. Travel is very important to me and maximizing my time (for me) must include travel and adventure. There are added challenges when traveling with a compromised immune system, as I'm sure you're well aware! Especially post COVID, I needed to come up with a strategy that would keep me relatively safe while allowing me to travel and interact with other cultures. It's just too important to put down, but I don't want to shorten my life any more than it already is.

It might be a little easier for me to pile my plate up with once-in-a-lifetime experiences because I can't sit still. All my life it has been about the next goal and the next challenge. I demand a lot from myself, and that is one of the reasons I've made it this far. Yes, it has helped me achieve success in business and at Vistage, and it motivated me to push myself when it really mattered, but I find it difficult to turn it off. That mindset is not always a great thing.

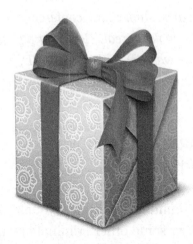

THE GIFT OF IMMEDIATE ACTION

All my life I've worked to improve, to just become a little better, a little wiser, a little stronger every day. Funny how mindset changes. Now, the goal of all my activities is to "prolong" my life. That's the word the doctors use, the literature uses, and, therefore, I will use. Prolonging life means to me having a good life for the rest of my life. It means to continue to live my mission. It means to appreciate every moment, every interaction, and every person I touch. It means not being defined by the harshness of chemo, but to persevere through the tough times and make each day as normal as possible.

It does not mean living well into my eighties or having the luxury of putting off important vacations or conversations. I think a lot about maximizing the time I have. There are about eight clients that I continue to meet with. These men have had relatively successful lives and are in strong financial positions. Our discussions revolve around three talking points for the rest of their lives:

1. How to facilitate and mentor an effective transition of both their business and their family values to the next generation of leaders
2. How to maximize the effectiveness of their time and treasure to have the greatest impact on our world
3. How to ensure they have a good life for the rest of their lives

Regarding number three, the conservative estimate that we use for the length of someone's active life is around eighty years. Therefore, those who are as old as I am, have thirteen good summers left. Even for those of us without incurable cancer, the need to maximize every day is undeniable. I, on the other hand, have one good summer at a time left and I don't even know if I'm guaranteed to have that. I choose to maximize my time starting with today.

CHAPTER TEN

2022

Happy New Year! The odds were against me living this long, but I continue to thrive and live an amazing life. Teresa and I vacationed in Hawaii right before Christmas. There was something about the islands that made me feel alive and grateful for every moment. During the trip, I read a book called *Chasing Daylight* written by Eugene O'Kelly. He was CEO of KPMG and was surprised when his doctor informed him that he had ninety days to live. He decided to write about his experience to provide a roadmap for those following him with similar diagnoses. He ended up passing close to the estimated ninety days and his wife wrote the final chapter in the book.

So much of what he wrote mirrored my feelings and outlook on cancer. Here are three examples:

1. He saw the diagnosis as a blessing because he had time to appreciate all the gifts this life had given him and was able to focus on only things that he felt were important to him during his last days.
2. He became very aware of creating and appreciating "perfect moments" as they occurred in his life. Before

his diagnosis, he might have seen one or two perfect moments a year. After diagnosis, he was able to appreciate many perfect moments each day. I also found that I experienced many perfect moments each day; holding hands while walking with Teresa and sharing intimate thoughts, watching the sun set as a whale breached on the horizon, waking, and snuggling for an extra ten minutes. The list goes on.

3. Letting people know how much he appreciated what they meant to his life. He made four lists based on impact and closeness and came up with 1,000 people he wanted to acknowledge. He then went on to contact them via email, letter, phone call, or in-person. This was something I thought about a lot. I stopped myself because of the limiting belief that people will think I am giving up. I planned to rethink this belief.

In the last chapter, I mentioned that I had a pain under my right rib cage. What I failed to mention was that I took a fall the month before that and landed hard on that area. It turned out the pain was not from new cancer or growth in my existing cancer. Apparently, I fractured my rib when I fell and had a partially collapsed lung.

I began the year with an MRI scheduled on my brain just to make sure the cancer had not returned there. This was a standard follow-up to my original brain tumor, and I did not expect to see any new cancer there. December 22 was the three-year anniversary of my first symptoms. What a blessing to know that I continue to thrive three years later.

A wonderful friend passed away from cancer and a long-term friend of my wife's was recently diagnosed. I was so ignorant of how prevalent and devastating cancer could be before my diagnosis! I keep having people I love and care for diagnosed and struggling or passing away. I have to say it again, cancer sucks!

BAD NEWS

I received the results of my MRI, and it appears the information is not good. We wouldn't know what that meant until we spoke with my oncologist, but I wanted to capture my emotions along the way. I quickly moved from sadness to acceptance with anticipation for more information and a plan of action.

The following is what was written by the MRI analyst:

IMPRESSION:
1. Compared to 8/20/2021, new focus of restricted diffusion with associated enhancement measuring up to 5 mm within the right precentral gyrus, suspicious for recurrence.
2. New nonspecific trace wispy enhancement within the adjacent right postcentral gyrus.

I was reading this as a new mass in my brain. I was stunned. I had a hard time speaking to Teresa to let her know what the report said. My eyes welled up and my body went numb, as I sat in stunned silence. I remained in a shocked state for several hours. After that, I found acceptance. Whatever it meant, I couldn't change it so I decided to move forward as I would any other day. I did send a note to my brain surgeon asking him to review the results and discuss with my oncologist before our next meeting.

I thought a lot about what this meant for Teresa and me going forward.

- How would it change the choices we were making about our time and my treatment?
- What did we need to do to maximize every moment?

There was so much unknown, I was sure I was putting the cart before the horse. But I couldn't hide from where my brain was taking me. We would take each step as it came starting with more information at the next doctor's visit. As I write, I am sitting on our patio in Mexico overlooking the ocean. There is no room for unhappiness in such a beautiful spot.

TEMPORARY RELIEF

The problem with a patient reviewing scan results without discussing with the doctor first is that the patient has a limited understanding of the problem. I emailed one doctor and called another one. The response from the first doctor summed it up pretty well:

"The CT chest looks stable, so the lung mass looks just fine. The MRI brain does show a single, small lesion. It is not clear if this lesion is a new lesion, a recurrent lesion of the previously treatment mass in 2019, or delayed radiation changes. For now, if you have no other symptoms (which I would expect since the lesion is so small), I suggest just repeating the MRI brain in about one month to look for any changes. Depending on any changes, we can make further decisions about the next steps. I'll order the repeat MRI for next month."

The scan caused quite an emotional roller coaster. My dreams were filled with memories of my youth. I thought about who impacted me the most and how they impacted me. There was a great deal of joy in those memories as they popped up in my dreams. It was fun thinking about so many experiences and people I had not thought of for years. The surprising thing for me was that I did not recall recent memories during these dreams. I even tried to force the issue but kept going back to my early days.

I would not say I was on an emotional high after learning of the doctor's cautious optimism because we still had to wait until the next scan to confirm his feelings. I would say that a weight has been lifted off my shoulders. Teresa and I gave each other a big hug and kiss afterwards. I was sure her burden lifted significantly as well.

JANUARY 21, 2022

The following post from my blog clearly demonstrates the emotional turmoil I experienced periodically throughout this journey.

"I broke my fibula and was sitting around in a cast trying to make the best of it. I broke it playing golf. I hit my drive down a slope and as I walked to the ball...slip, pop, ouch, oh crap! The break was down by the ankle in two spots. I was so frustrated and disappointed. All I was trying to do was live a good life while living with lung cancer. Was that too much to ask? Instead, obstacles kept launching themselves in my path."

First it was COVID limiting all travel and social interaction. Then it was radiation on my lungs that kept me from doing much of anything for two months. After that it was radiation pneumonitis that sidelined me for three months and then the cure, prednisone, sidelined me another two months. And now, a broken leg had me out of the game. We were supposed to head to the Bahamas but cancelled that.

MORE BAD NEWS

We knew this day would come. For the past week and a half, I had a dull headache and a bit of dizziness. The feeling was exacerbated by multiple bouts of vertigo. If you have not experienced vertigo, it's like standing in the middle of a merry-go-round while all the characters whiz by at high speed. However, in my case the pictures on the walls and the furniture would whiz by. I literally had to grab something or immediately sit down to keep from falling.

I shared this information with my oncologist who felt it was pertinent to move up my next MRI to get an immediate look at my brain. I had the MRI Monday. The next night, we were sitting down to dinner with some good friends when the doctor called. We had a nice, calm conversation where he explained that I had two spots in my brain that had grown a little since my last MRI 30 days ago. He further noted that I had swelling in the brain causing my headache, dizziness, and vertigo. He said the ball was now in my brain doctor's court and I needed to talk with him about next steps.

I hung up the phone and turned to Teresa to share the news. We looked at each other with tears in our eyes and hugged. Fortunately, we recovered quickly and had a wonderful dinner with our friends. On the other hand, we did not sleep well that night as thoughts of "what's next" spun through our heads.

I received a note from the brain doctor, and he was not overly concerned. The lesions were small, and he was not convinced they were significant. He ordered an analysis overlapping my original MRI from three years ago with the current MRI to determine if the lesions were new or related to the first. He felt the lesions were too small to deal with for the time being and ordered a new MRI sixty days later. He said he had no concerns about travel (we were flying to Bogota on Saturday).

EMOTIONAL CANCER BUNGEE CORD

Having cancer put me through an emotional bungee cord. The first diagnosis had me dive down to where I thought death was inches away, gasping for breath, wondering if I would stop on time, and feeling totally out of control. Then the discussions with doctors and medical plans had me springing back to positivity and hope and a brighter day.

Setbacks and unwanted results loosened the pull of hope as I rapidly sped towards despair. Then again, the strategy changed, and I sprang back up to see a brighter day. Down and up I went as time passed, each swing diminishing in arch. I assumed that, like a bungee cord, a point would come when the ups and downs would come to an end and I would find myself suspended at the end of the rope.

At that point, I would either be pulled back up to join the others who are awaiting their turn, or, I would be lowered to the canyon floor where I would peacefully end my journey as others have before me.

NECESSITY OF VULNERABILITY

A lot of cancer patients don't want anyone to know what they are going through. They ask their loved ones to keep it to themselves and allow very few people to join or observe their journey. I cannot speak to their motivations as I do not understand their approach. I can only speak to the strength, joy, hope and love Teresa and I get from vulnerability. By sharing my journey, I receive many rewards and offer a few gifts as well. Through expression, I better understand my feelings around my journey. I allow Teresa to share her hopes and fears openly around others when I am not present. I provide an opportunity for those in my community to feel and understand their emotions around cancer, to express their love for me, Teresa, and others in their life, and to develop their own strategies for current and future encounters with cancer. And, most importantly, I provide an opportunity for others to wrap their arms around Teresa, my sister, my mother, and others who are hurting because of my cancer journey.

If you have cancer or any other disease, I encourage you to open up to others in your community. Give them the opportunity to share your journey and express their love— it will be a gift for both of you. If you have a friend with cancer or know someone who is experiencing some other medical challenge, I encourage you to seek opportunities to engage with them. What I appreciate is when friends listen and empathize with my journey. What may not be helpful is when they prescribe, suggest, or "should" on me. Just be an active empathetic listener and you will be appreciated.

THOUGHTS ABOUT LOVE

I have always been someone who openly expressed my love for others in my life whether it be the romantic love I feel for Teresa, the familial love I have for siblings and close friends, or the love I feel for all others that cross my path throughout my life. The other side of the coin has changed dramatically. I struggled to receive love as I had convinced myself that I had not earned the right to be loved. Since my diagnosis, I've learned that being loved and having others express that love is probably the most fulfilling experience, and that it's not all about me.

First, love is a gift that I've learned to graciously accept as it fills me with self-worth, hope, and gratitude. Second, giving love is joyful for the giver. To share feelings and let another know they are valued is empowering. I have seen time and time again that by letting other people know I care for them, I too am filled with love and joy. I believe that the outpouring of love I'm experiencing has been cathartic and joyful for the giver as well.

We met with the doctor, and he said I remained "unremarkable." He said I was one of those unique cases where the chemo was really working long term. He also agreed with my brain specialist, in that he was not too concerned about the spots on the MRI. He said there were lots of conditions that could have caused the spots to show up in the exact same place as my original tumors that are not cancer.

If the spots were somewhere different, he would have been concerned. We would wait for the results of my April MRI to see if anything changes. Teresa and I also pushed to get back on Keytruda (immunotherapy). Since the chemo was working so well, the doctor still wanted to keep Keytruda in his back pocket for if/when things get worse.

THOUGHTS ON MY LAST DAYS ON EARTH

My cousin texted me to inform me that her husband was coming home to die. They would provide in-home hospice care for "comfort only" as he slowly passes. A couple of realizations hit me. First, I assumed he was ready to go and was embracing the love and comfort of family and the peace of being in his own home. Second, the real pain was only waiting for those he would have to leave behind. There is such a finality to death. This would be the last time my cousin and her family would get to see him, to embrace him, and to share their love with him. It was heartbreaking to see and feel their pain. Teresa and I have felt that pain every night since I received her text as we have cried for my cousin, her family, and for the eventuality of my final moments.

I didn't just hurt for her husband, I hurt for my cousin and Teresa. They would no longer have their best friend, their confidant, or their lover. They won't have the person they have shared special moments with for so many years. There will be a time when they turn and talk to us, and we won't be there. I cried as I thought about Teresa's solo journey in life when she is forced to move forward without me. I want to hold her so tightly, not for me but for her. I felt so powerless in helping, comforting, and embracing her.

Something else I was thinking about over the past three years was what I would want in my last days, when I too am in hospice care. I will want my wife to hold me, to crawl into bed with me, and to hold my hand constantly. I'd want anyone who came to visit me to share stories of good times together, embarrassing moments, and crazy adventures. More importantly for me, I'd want anyone and everyone who visited to share stories and words I've expressed that influenced their lives, that even today they think about at opportune moments.

As I'm writing this book, I continue to have conversations with Teresa and how this is impacting both of us. Recently, we shared that we both have been walking around the house trying to find the best place to put the hospice bed when the time arises. What a crazy thing to be thinking about while I continue to thrive. The good news is that we chose the exact same spot for the exact same reason.

UNEXPECTED RECOGNITION

I was so humbled and honored that the organization I've spent the past 20 years with (Vistage) decided to create an annual legacy award for newer Vistage Chairs called the Les Whitney Perseverance Award. This annual award will be given to one individual who has overcome adversity and challenge during their first few years to build a successful Vistage practice. Following is what Vistage wrote about the award:

> "Les Whitney began his Vistage journey as a member in 2000. During that time, he recognized the significant role a Chair plays in the lives of leaders and decided

Chairing would be his next step. In 2004, Les completed Chair onboarding and began his career as a Vistage Chair. Over the years, he achieved numerous awards and recognitions including Rookie of the Year, multiple Chair Excellence Awards, a lifetime Master Chair recognition, and most recently designated as a Chair Emeritus.

Looking to serve the Chair community further, in 2008, Les made a significant impact by onboarding new Chairs throughout the country, helping each of them achieve their goal of starting their own Chair practice. Les believes that new Chairs are key to helping new members and their companies succeed and has never looked at another Chair as a competitor. His motto is "If they are successful, we are all successful."

Over the years, Les has had to overcome his own adversity, including a significant cancer diagnosis in 2019. His persistence, determination, and positive outlook have been an inspiration for the entire Vistage community."

What an honor!

MARCH 2022

I'm tired of cancer.

Actually, I'm fed up with it. Not just what it is doing to me, but the impact it has had on so many friends and family members. Cancer just seems to show up everywhere in such an ugly way.

My cousin's husband passed away. Cancer was so unfair to him and his family. He was diagnosed around Thanksgiving and was gone on February 24th. Everything happened so fast that there was limited time for the family to adjust and prepare for life without him. He was in and out of hospitals and/or devastated by the pain of the cancer and the pain of the treatments. To make matters worse, he wasn't allowed many visitors when hospitalized because of COVID. I don't know if he and his family ever had the opportunity to talk about life, death, and what was next for those he left behind. It was another reminder to me that these conversations are important regardless of one's current health.

One of our closest friends, Kathy, succumbed to her cancer. Kathy was such a strong and courageous woman who made sure she lived her life in the way she wanted as fully as she possibly could given the pain from the cancer and the debilitating impact radiation and chemotherapy had on her body. Her treatments caused huge swings in her physicality, ability to enjoy life, and even ability to communicate. It reminded me of my bungee cord analogy. When she was healthy, she travelled to spend time with her daughters and grandchildren.

In fact, one daughter told me that she spent more time with her mom in the past year than she did in the prior five years. She didn't only visit, she communicated. They talked about how wonderful their lives together had been. They talked about the hopes and dreams for the future for her daughters and grandchildren. She talked about her hopes for her husband, their father, after she was gone. In other words, she communicated everything she felt needed to be communicated before she passed. I could not think of a more precious gift for those you leave behind.

Recently, another friend informed me that she was diagnosed with multiple myeloma, a blood-based cancer.

She would begin treatment in a couple of weeks and the prognosis was good. It irritated me that another friend had to suffer the devastating effects of chemo, radiation and, in her case, a bone marrow transplant. As I was writing this book, I reviewed my CaringBridge posts and the comments from my followers. I came across a comment she had written about cancer, strength in how one could respond, and how inspirational I had been to her. I copied her note and sent it to her as if it were my own only adding the attribution to her at the end. She called me in tears and informed me that that was the most love she had felt from a friend since her journey began.

APRIL 2022

I was finally out of the cast and boot from my broken ankle and very nearly back to 100%. But that was the end of the good news. I was so tired all the time. The chemo was just doing a number on me again. When we went out, I was constantly fighting exhaustion. Not that anyone would notice as I pushed through the fatigue, but once home I was down for the count. I struggled with motivation to do anything productive, even reading a book or playing the ukulele felt like a major endeavor. It was such a burden to rely on self-talk to psych myself up to partake in the simplest of tasks.

It was weighing heavily on me that my life was controlled by cancer, chemo, doctors' appointments, and my physical limitations caused by it all. I was tired of my nose running 24/7 because of the chemo. I was tired of feeling a little out of sorts every day. I was tired of constantly having to "overcome" all that was going on with me and around me. I was tired of being tired.

Confident this state of mind would pass quickly, I chalked it up to a product of losing friends and family and being limited by a broken ankle piled on top of all the crap that was cancer and its treatment. It appeared that once every six months I fell into a short-lived funk and today was that day. Such is the up and down bungee cord journey of a cancer patient.

I did turn around rather quickly after about five days, even after we were informed that Teresa lost another close friend to cancer just a month after it was discovered. It is truly awful how often cancer shows up and how quickly it can take loved ones from us.

I met with my doctor in mid-2022 to review the MRI of my brain and CT scan of my torso that was taken two weeks prior. The lesions on the brain remained but were unchanged. This likely meant there was no new cancer, and the spots were just a reaction to my original SRS surgery. Yippee! The CT scan remained mostly unremarkable. The CT technician did notice an enlargement of my adrenal gland and a 10mm spot. The doctor and I compared the last four CT scans to see if there was any change and we couldn't see one. We decided to do an MRI of that area the following week just to make sure, but also to create a baseline to compare to future MRIs.

My colleagues at Vistage presented me with a trip to San Diego when I retired. Teresa and I grew up and met in San Diego. The highlight of the trip was the Seven Bridges walk. It went through various neighborhoods and crossed seven old walking bridges that were built around 1910. We walked past the hospital where Teresa was born, her high school, Athena's high school, the place we met, the place we would meet in the morning and walk hand in hand to work, our favorite breakfast restaurant, and so much more. Since we chose to walk from our hotel, we ended up walking thirteen miles that day. In fact, we've walked at least six miles a day for the past two weeks. I was over my broken ankle.

After the next chemo session, we were off to Palm Springs for a week. The following chemo would be May 20, then we were scheduled to fly to Iceland on May 25 followed by Boulder Colorado in June, nothing yet for July and August and then a train trip in the Canadian Rockies on the Rocky Mountaineer in September. We were also looking forward to Japan in November. My doctor informed us that he lives vicariously through us...not bad for a cancer patient.

We've been at this for three and a half years. The longer we go with no change, the more likely it is that we will continue to thrive.

TESTIMONIAL: MOHAMMAD KHAN

Mohammad is another Vistage colleague who made a big impression on me. I was excited to learn that I was just as instrumental in his life! Here is his story:

I was a member of Les's professional team. I met him a few years back. He came into the office, and I was instantaneously drawn to him. He was just a wonderful guy who showed up in his wine shirt (a tropical themed button down with pictures of wine on it). At the time, I was thinking about joining some executive network, and I was interviewing with a couple. I met Les in person, and I just got a good vibe with him. Ever since then, he's been probably the most critical mentor figure or coach in my professional career outside of my wife. He means the world to me.

I'm an attorney. At the time, I was also the chief operating officer of a CPA and law firm. I broke off and started my own legal practice and Les was the driving force in that decision.

When I decided to make the move away from my firm, it was something I was toying with for a little bit. It was probably one of the times I was the most vulnerable professionally. And I was looking for support and guidance. So, I called Les up and said, "Hey, this is what's going on." He immediately dropped everything to start giving me advice. Every step of the way, all the way to when I gave my resignation letter to starting my own practice, he was there. I think the day I gave my resignation letter, he texted me in the morning to say, "I'm with you, stay strong." I don't know that I could have made such a drastic move from my comfortable job as CEO to starting my own practice without his guidance and support.

At the time, I hadn't lost anyone to cancer but during this process, I lost my mom. It really was a strange feeling, having somebody so close and someone I cared about both going through the same thing. So, I was broken up about it. But the way he continued to show up, he was always himself. You wouldn't even think that this guy had stage IV cancer. It got me to reprioritize things and helped me make certain professional decisions, in terms of how I would prioritize family time. And living every day like you mean it, that was an important lesson that I learned from Les.

I follow him on his blog and there's always little nuggets of wisdom that come out. It's helped me adapt and appreciate everything a lot more. I think what I learned from Les is that the more you give to others, the more you get. He cares so much about other people, and he gives to so many people. And I think it's because he's a great guy, but he also gets so much back from it. It's that culture of service and his commitment to others that really inspired me to be a better person myself.

LESSONS LEARNED: "THIS TOO SHALL END"

In my situation, I am going to have to put up with chemo for the rest of my life. No matter how long that is, doctors have assured me that I will be undergoing treatment in one form or another until it is no longer successful in containing my cancer. To bring myself around from the "dying every month" mentality, I like to tell myself that *"this too shall end."*

Nutrition and exercise are the keys to feeling better no matter what I'm going through. From what I read, cancer patients are done in by the chemo and their inability to function, to eat, and to take care of themselves while getting the treatment. I will not allow that to happen to me. I will eat even when I don't want to, I will exercise even when I don't want to, and I will continue to work and be an effective presence for my friends and family even when I don't want to. I will do all these things because that is what it is going to take to win. I've always had the ability to push through pain. That experience was the precursor to my fight with incurable cancer.

It's now quite common for me to feel like I have a low-grade flu. It is a nuisance, but nothing I can't handle. I am still adjusting to this because even after three and a half years and 60 chemo treatments, it is so different from my normal, healthy self. Historically, I have plowed through sickness and injuries as if they did not exist. My body and my mind have not figured out how to plow through cancer so I am learning to slow down, take what I can from each day, and rest when I need to rest. I think it is harder on me mentally than physically because I keep judging myself, expecting to be tougher and stronger. I'm getting lots of good advice to go with the flow, to rest, to allow my body to dictate my needs, and I believe I am doing a good job of following that advice...just not without judgement.

Proof that "this too shall end" can be found in my friends. I've been surprised at all the cancer survival stories from people we know and meet. Recently, our friend Jay shared that he has been in remission for ten years from two types of rare, deadly cancer.

Jay was kind enough to share his story, which mirrors mine in some ways. When first diagnosed, his doctor muttered under his breath that Jay should have been dead six months ago. He gave Jay very little chance to survive.

One thing about the statistics of cancer survival is that, with the uniqueness of each individual, the statistics don't mean much. When Jay was first diagnosed, his chance of survival was very low. Now that he *is* a survivor, he pretty much has a 50/50 chance of surviving each year as it comes. It is nice to think that the longer I survive, the odds of continuing to survive improve.

Jay shared a final note about a friend of his who received that same stage IV lung cancer diagnosis as mine. He has been undergoing chemo every three weeks for the past six years and continues to thrive. His cancer has not grown and remains controlled if he continues the chemo. His attitude is that he can suffer through five days of yuckiness every three weeks as long as he thrives during the remaining sixteen days. Apparently, he is traveling extensively during his "between times" and making sure to connect with friends and family. He is even investigating getting chemo in Europe for one of his sessions so that he can extend a trip to five weeks.

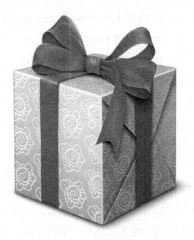

THE GIFT OF PERFECT MOMENTS

In this chapter, I mentioned the book *Chasing Daylight*. In it the author shared his thoughts about "perfect moments."

Throughout my life, I have had my share of perfect moments. Seeing my wife walking down the aisle on our wedding day. Moving into our first house. Standing in front of the pyramids of Giza imagining that Alexander the Great stood exactly where I was standing. The list goes on and on, but these perfect moments were limited to a few per year.

Now that I am embracing perfect moments as they come, I experience a few each day. They may be a belly laugh from Teresa over something I've said, taking a turn on a walk and discovering a magical hidden garden, an "aha" moment during a conversation, or a smile from a child in a playground. The list of perfect moments goes on and on. Our smiles are broad and our hearts are filled as we pause for a few seconds and experience the moment.

Perfect moments are everywhere, and it only takes two actions to keep them present in your life. First, be present to your surroundings. Put away the phone, and clear your mind of thoughts outside of your current environment. Be open to what life has to offer. Second, take a few seconds to accept and appreciate the moment. If you are with someone, stop and share that this was a perfect moment. If you are alone, be grateful for life's gift.

Stop! Breath! Was reading about this gift a perfect moment?

TESTIMONIAL: TERESA

Teresa needs no introduction. If you've read to this point in the book, you know that she is my wife of 37 years. Here is another perspective of our journey in her words. Perhaps it will give you a different lens to see things through.

When I met Les, we were both working for San Diego Gas and Electric Company, and we were both runners. Our building did not have showers, so all the people that ran or exercised over their lunch breaks would cross the street to the city of San Diego's facilities to shower in their concourse building. I would see him as I was going in and he was leaving. I was taken by how friendly he was and how he always had the biggest smile on his face.

We had a common friend, Mike Feori. Mike and I were coordinating the 10k race for our company, and Les was his buddy. I was 29, and he was 26 at the time. He was just as hyper as he is now. He just couldn't stop moving and doing. I mean, even to this day if he is sitting with you, his leg is moving.

He has always been a very confident and outgoing person. When I met him, he was volunteering for Special Olympics, coordinating the largest meet of the year. He was involved in so many different things in business, in the community, and completing his master's degree.

Les is one of the most caring and open individuals I've ever met. He truly wants to make a difference in people's lives. And he says what he thinks always. I often say he has no filter.

He is also incredibly honest. I mean, if somebody gives him the wrong change, even down to 20 cents or something, he'll go back and make it right. I remember when we were dating, I told him that somebody was offering to sell me this camera at a great deal.

He said, "Teresa, if that's that good of a deal, it's probably stolen. And you don't want to support anything like that." I never thought of it that way.

Once he left San Diego Gas and Electric Company, he went into international business. And he started traveling. By that time, we were married, so that was the start of my travel. It opened a whole new world, to see how people live in other places and realizing that people are just people no matter where they are from.

We went to Africa once and went into the Kabira slums. We saw a whole community, almost like a city of people that were living in shacks made of any material they could find. They had no infrastructure support from the Kenyan government. They created their own security force outside of the police in Nairobi, and they had these little businesses in their shacks. They had to walk forever to get clean water. It was an eye-opener.

Through travel together, we have learned to be grateful for all that we have been blessed with. We realize that every day that we wake up is a good day. In his career as a CEO of companies, he made such important decisions. And then to see him at a family get-together playing with the kids on a skateboard, I thought, oh my God, look at you. You're just a big kid.

My mother passed away from cancer when she was eighty-four. That was my first experience with cancer. My sister passed away from pancreatic cancer shortly after. Like Les says, it seems like we're losing more and more friends and family to the illness the further along on this journey we go.

It's his day-to-day struggles after chemo treatments that impact me the most. We are trying to squeeze in as much living as we can in the time that we have. Not knowing how much time we have is difficult.

Even though Les's cancer is my number one priority, I still find time to be active in the community. This is important to me. I'm on the board of a lady's golf club. I just completed my term as president of our local garden club. We raise money for scholarships and children's activities in schools through our Rotary Club. I also belong to a group called San Clemente Village, where I volunteer and drive people to doctor appointments. I take them grocery shopping, so that elderly or people with disabilities can stay in their homes.

I think Les is writing this book for himself as well as other people. It's cathartic for him. But his blog has helped so many people already, it's amazing. People that have cancer and people that have friends or family that have cancer have all felt, seen, heard, and been impacted by the experiences Les shares. I love it because I get to read what he is thinking. Sometimes, it's hard to read topics about death and how difficult it has all been. We don't always talk about those tough times until after Les expresses himself through writing.

That's one thing that is very different from me. I am a very private person. This is very hard for me to share my thoughts *here. I think it's good for me that he's so positive all the time. But it's painful that our life as we planned it, is not happening. He would always tease me and say, "I can't wait to grow old with you." Now I don't know if that's going to happen.*

He talks about what is going on and shares his struggles with others. I'm very good at suppressing. I just tell myself: I don't need to deal with that now. So, when people say, "what can I do for you? Do you need help?" My response is, "No, not right now. I'm sure there'll be a time in the future, but I'm handling things well right now." I have Les promise me every morning that he won't leave until ten years from today. But I know mentally he plans for three years.

I think when you have adversity in your life, you just face it. One day at a time, you just don't have a choice. So, I make the most of it and move on. Move forward and move on. Just one day at a time.

CONCLUSION

The word "conclusion" is somewhat misleading. As of the writing of this book, I am still thriving and living my life to the fullest. I've had 63 chemo sessions and many more planned. I am still around for the amazing little moments and still griping about the recovery periods I am forced to go through on a three-week basis.

I want to thank all the people who were kind enough to give testimonials. Your words validate all the work I put into presenting a positive attitude and give me more joy than you could possibly imagine! I am lucky in many ways to have been able to experience such love, friendship, and support from hundreds of amazing people.

To my Vistage colleagues, I would like to say that I have enjoyed every meeting, every retreat, every conference I have ever attended. You do incredible work, and you affect the lives of so many people in a truly positive way. No matter how long I am with you, I want you to know that you gave me as much inspiration as I could ever hope to share with you.

To my friends and family who filled my time and travels with camaraderie, I want to thank you for opening your homes and your hearts to Teresa and me. We benefited immensely from your generosity and had many great adventures together!

There are no words that I can commit to paper that would adequately sum up my feelings for the most important woman in my life. I am determined to spend what time I have left making sure Teresa knows how I feel, so I will be brief here. I LOVE YOU! Thank you for spending your life with me, for holding my hand up to the end. I never could have achieved half of what I was able to without your generosity, kindness, and attention. I wish I could continue to live if only so that I wouldn't have to leave you. It is my greatest regret and the hardest thing I have had to deal with throughout this cancer nightmare.

I am going to leave a few blank pages at the end of this book. It is my hope that you can fill them up with your memories, with stories that haven't happened yet, and things you would like to remember about me and our time together.

None of us know how much time we have left.

Don't squander a second.

Take care of each other.

Make that phone call you've been putting off.

Send that note card to someone you've been thinking of.

Smile with no reason.

Whatever it is that you dream of doing, do yourself and your loved ones a huge favor.

Put down this book and do it.

Do it now.

Made in United States
North Haven, CT
07 February 2023

32209372R00134